THE COMPLETE FOODS LISTS FOR KIDNEY DISEASE

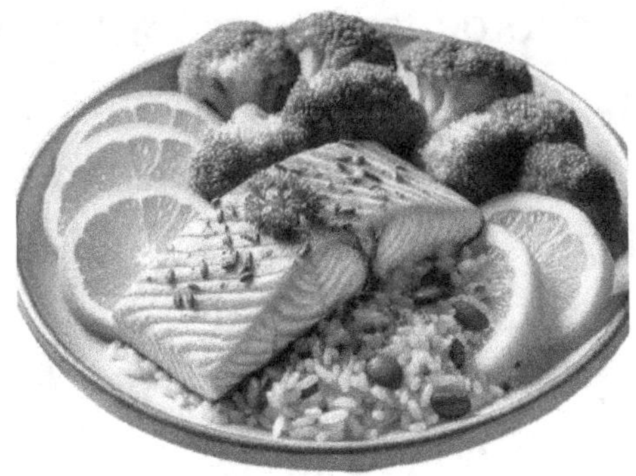

Detailed Guide to Kidney-Friendly Recipes, Providing 1000+ Foods with Sodium, Potassium, and Phosphorus Contents and Practical Guidelines for Managing CKD

Tina Feldman

Table of Content

Introduction...5

Understanding Your Kidneys and Chronic Kidney Disease
(CKD) 7

    The Vital Role of Your Kidneys.............................7

    What is Chronic Kidney Disease (CKD)? 9

    Recognizing the Signs and Symptoms of CKD 11

    Causes and Risk Factors for Developing CKD...............14

    Stages of Chronic Kidney Disease.........................17

PART 2 21

Making Smart Food Choices for Kidney Health 21

    Embracing Whole and Minimally Processed Foods............21

    A Guide to Kidney-Friendly Whole Foods and their Benefits
....24

    Eating Low-Glycemic and Anti-Inflammatory Foods 29

    Minimizing High-Glycemic and Inflammatory Foods 33

Part 3 37

Managing Diabetes and Kidney Health Together...............37

    Demystifying the Glycemic Index 37

    The Power of a Low-Glycemic Diet for Your Health.........41

    Making a Low-Glycemic Lifestyle Work for You 44

Part 4: 48

    The Essential Potassium, Phosphorus, and Sodium Counter.48

    Baked Goods..48

    Beans, Lentils, and Kidney-Friendly Choices.............54

    Beverages..62

    Breakfast Cereals 70

Dairy and Dairy Alternatives 77

Dressings, Fats, and Oils..85

Fast Food Products...93

Fruits and Fruit Products..101

Fish and Seafood...109

Grains and Pasta...117

Meat 125

Nuts and Seeds...133

Spices and Herbs..141

Vegetables and Vegetable Products................................149

Part 5 157

25 Healthy and Delicious Renal friendly recipes for CKD......157

Soup and stew 157

Side dishes 162

Mains 167

Salads..173

Snack and Appetizer 178

Cooking Techniques to Reduce Sodium and Phosphorus in Meals..183

BONUS 1 186

30 days kidney diseases meals plan 186

BONUS 2: KIDNEY DISEASE MEAL TRACKER 212

....241

Conclusion 243

Introduction

Kidneys play a pivotal role as silent guardians, tirelessly filtering waste and maintaining a delicate balance within our bodies. When kidney disease disrupts this intricate dance, it necessitates a thoughtful reevaluation of dietary choices to support optimal well-being.

Welcome to "The Complete Foods Lists for Kidney Disease," a comprehensive guide designed to empower individuals facing the challenges of kidney health with knowledge about the foods that can promote healing, sustain vitality, and contribute to an improved quality of life.

As we embark on this journey, it is crucial to recognize the profound impact nutrition can have on kidney function. The intricate interplay between nutrients and kidney health underscores the importance of making informed decisions about what we consume. This guide aims to serve as a trustworthy companion, providing a meticulously curated selection of foods that align with the unique dietary needs of individuals grappling with kidney disease.

Within these pages, you will discover not just a list of foods but a holistic approach to nutrition tailored specifically for kidney health. Backed by the latest scientific insights, our curated lists encompass a spectrum of nutrients, flavors, and culinary options to cater to different tastes and dietary preferences.

Whether you are a seasoned cook or someone just beginning to navigate the intricacies of kidney-friendly eating, this guide is designed to be accessible, informative, and, above all, empowering.

In addition to presenting a comprehensive list of kidney-friendly foods, we will delve into the principles that guide these dietary recommendations. Understanding the rationale behind food choices empowers individuals to make informed decisions that resonate with their unique health journey. From managing protein intake and sodium levels to exploring the benefits of antioxidant-rich foods, this guide will equip you with the knowledge needed to make conscious and healthful dietary choices.

"Foods Lists for Kidney Disease" is more than a compilation of ingredients; it is a roadmap towards a nourished and vibrant life despite the challenges posed by kidney disease. As we navigate the terrain of nutrition and well-being, let this guide be a beacon of hope, providing the tools and insights needed to embrace a kidney-friendly lifestyle and embark on a journey towards renewed health.

Understanding Your Kidneys and Chronic Kidney Disease (CKD)

The Vital Role of Your Kidneys

The kidneys, two bean-shaped organs nestled discreetly in the lower back, are unsung heroes of the human body, quietly performing a multitude of essential functions that are paramount to our overall well-being. Understanding the intricate role these organs play in maintaining homeostasis and supporting vital bodily functions is crucial for appreciating their significance in the intricate dance of human physiology.

Filtration and Waste Removal:
The primary function of the kidneys is to filter and eliminate waste products and excess fluids from the blood, forming urine that is then expelled from the body. This critical process ensures the removal of toxins and metabolic by-products, preventing the accumulation of harmful substances within the bloodstream.

Fluid and Electrolyte Balance:
Kidneys maintain a delicate balance of fluids and electrolytes in the body. By selectively reabsorbing essential substances like sodium, potassium, and calcium, they regulate blood pressure, support nerve function, and contribute to the overall stability of bodily fluids.

Blood Pressure Regulation:
The kidneys play a pivotal role in controlling blood pressure by adjusting the volume of blood and releasing the enzyme renin. Renin acts on the angiotensin system to regulate blood vessel constriction and fluid balance, influencing blood pressure levels.

Red Blood Cell Production:
Erythropoietin, a hormone produced by the kidneys, stimulates the bone marrow to produce red blood cells. This process, known as erythropoiesis, ensures an adequate supply of oxygen-carrying red blood cells to tissues and organs, supporting overall oxygenation and energy metabolism.

Acid-Base Balance:
Kidneys help maintain the body's acid-base balance by excreting hydrogen ions and reabsorbing bicarbonate. This regulatory function is vital for ensuring the proper pH levels of bodily fluids, which, in turn, influence enzymatic activity and metabolic processes.

Vitamin D Activation:
The kidneys convert inactive vitamin D into its active form, which is essential for the absorption of calcium and phosphate in the intestines. This activation supports bone health and helps maintain the integrity of the skeletal system.

Glucose Regulation:
Kidneys contribute to glucose regulation by reabsorbing glucose back into the bloodstream, preventing its

excessive loss in urine. This function is particularly crucial during periods of fasting or low blood sugar

What is Chronic Kidney Disease (CKD)?

Chronic Kidney Disease, commonly abbreviated as CKD, is a progressive and irreversible condition characterized by the gradual loss of kidney function over an extended period. This condition poses a significant health challenge as the kidneys, vital organs responsible for various crucial functions in the body, experience a decline in their ability to filter waste products and maintain fluid and electrolyte balance. CKD is a global health concern affecting millions of people and is often asymptomatic in its early stages, making early detection and management crucial for mitigating its impact.

1. Stages of CKD:

CKD is classified into five stages, ranging from Stage 1 (mild kidney damage) to Stage 5 (end-stage renal disease or ESRD). Each stage represents a progressive decline in kidney function, with Stage 5 requiring renal replacement therapy, such as dialysis or kidney transplantation, for survival.

2. Common Causes:

CKD can result from various underlying conditions that impair kidney function. Diabetes and hypertension (high blood pressure) are leading causes of CKD, accounting for a substantial percentage of cases. Other causes include glomerulonephritis, polycystic kidney disease, urinary tract obstructions, and certain autoimmune diseases.

3. Symptoms and Diagnosis:

In its early stages, CKD often presents with minimal or no symptoms, making it challenging to detect. As the disease progresses, symptoms may include fatigue, swelling (edema), changes in urine output, increased or decreased frequency of urination, and difficulty concentrating. Diagnosis typically involves blood tests to assess kidney function, urine tests to check for the presence of protein and other abnormalities, and imaging studies.

4. Complications:

CKD is associated with a range of complications that can affect various organ systems. These include cardiovascular diseases, anemia, bone and mineral disorders, and an increased risk of infections. Additionally, CKD can contribute to the progression of other health conditions, further impacting overall well-being.

5. Management and Treatment:

Management of CKD involves slowing the progression of the disease, addressing its underlying causes, and managing associated complications. Lifestyle modifications, including dietary changes, regular exercise, and blood pressure control, play a crucial role.

Medications may be prescribed to manage specific symptoms and conditions associated with CKD.

6. Prevention:

Early detection and intervention are key to slowing the progression of CKD. Managing risk factors such as diabetes, hypertension, and maintaining a healthy lifestyle through balanced nutrition and regular physical activity contribute significantly to prevention.

Recognizing the Signs and Symptoms of CKD

Chronic Kidney Disease (CKD) is often referred to as a "silent" condition, as it may progress slowly without manifesting noticeable symptoms in its early stages. However, understanding the signs and symptoms that may emerge as CKD advances is crucial for early detection and effective management. Here's an overview of the key indicators to be aware of:

1. Changes in Urination:

Increased Urination (Polyuria): CKD can lead to an increased urge to urinate, especially at night.
Decreased Urination (Oliguria): In some cases, CKD may result in reduced urine output, indicating impaired kidney function.

2. Fluid Retention and Swelling (Edema):

As the kidneys struggle to regulate fluid balance, excess fluid can accumulate, leading to swelling in the legs, ankles, feet, and sometimes the face.

3. Fatigue and Weakness:

CKD can cause anemia due to reduced production of erythropoietin, a hormone that stimulates red blood cell production. Anemia, in turn, can result in fatigue, weakness, and decreased energy levels.

4. Changes in Urine Characteristics:

Foamy Urine: Excessive protein in the urine, known as proteinuria, may cause urine to appear foamy.
Blood in Urine (Hematuria): CKD can lead to blood in the urine, which may be visible or detected through laboratory tests.

5. Persistent Itching (Pruritus):

The accumulation of waste products in the bloodstream, especially urea, can cause persistent itching.

6. High Blood Pressure (Hypertension):

CKD and hypertension often coexist, and one can exacerbate the other. Elevated blood pressure can further damage the kidneys, creating a harmful cycle.

7. Difficulty Concentrating and Mental Fog:

Impaired kidney function can lead to a buildup of toxins in the bloodstream, affecting cognitive function and concentration.

8. Loss of Appetite and Weight Loss:

CKD may result in a reduced appetite, accompanied by unintentional weight loss.

9. Muscle Cramps and Twitching:

Electrolyte imbalances associated with CKD can lead to muscle cramps and twitching.

10. Bone and Joint Problems:

CKD can disrupt the balance of calcium and phosphorus in the body, contributing to bone and joint problems.

11. Shortness of Breath:

As CKD progresses, fluid accumulation and anemia can lead to shortness of breath, especially during physical exertion.

12. Increased Frequency of Infections:

Weakened immune function and impaired response to infections can result from CKD.

Note: It is important to note that the severity and combination of symptoms can vary among individuals, and some people with CKD may remain asymptomatic until the disease has advanced. Regular health check-ups, especially for those with risk factors such as diabetes and hypertension, are essential for early detection and proactive management of CKD.

Causes and Risk Factors for Developing CKD

Chronic Kidney Disease (CKD) can arise from a variety of underlying causes, and its development is often influenced by a combination of genetic, environmental, and lifestyle factors. Understanding the potential triggers and risk factors is essential for both prevention and early intervention. Here's a detailed exploration of the causes and risk factors associated with CKD:

1. Diabetes Mellitus:

Cause: Diabetes is a leading cause of CKD. Persistent high levels of blood glucose can damage the blood vessels in the kidneys, impairing their function over time.
Risk Factor: Individuals with Type 1 or Type 2 diabetes are at an increased risk of developing CKD.

2. Hypertension (High Blood Pressure):

Cause: Uncontrolled high blood pressure is a major contributor to CKD. Elevated pressure within the blood vessels of the kidneys can lead to damage over time.
Risk Factor: Chronic hypertension is a significant risk factor for CKD, and individuals with high blood pressure should monitor and manage it to prevent kidney damage.

3. Glomerulonephritis:

Cause: Glomerulonephritis involves inflammation of the glomeruli, the small filtering units in the kidneys. This inflammation can result from infections,

autoimmune diseases, or other immune system-related disorders.
Risk Factor: Individuals with a history of infections, autoimmune conditions, or a family history of glomerulonephritis may be at an increased risk.

4. Polycystic Kidney Disease (PKD):

Cause: PKD is a genetic disorder characterized by the formation of fluid-filled cysts within the kidneys, leading to structural damage and impaired function.
Risk Factor: Individuals with a family history of PKD have an increased risk of inheriting the condition.

5. Urinary Tract Obstructions:

Cause: Obstructions in the urinary tract, such as kidney stones or tumors, can impede the flow of urine, leading to kidney damage.
Risk Factor: Individuals with a history of recurrent urinary tract infections, kidney stones, or structural abnormalities may be at an increased risk.

6. Recurrent Kidney Infections:

Cause: Repeated kidney infections can cause scarring and damage to the kidneys, contributing to the development of CKD.
Risk Factor: Individuals with a history of frequent or inadequately treated kidney infections are at an increased risk.

7. Systemic Diseases:

Cause: Certain systemic conditions, such as lupus, multiple myeloma, and vasculitis, can affect the kidneys and lead to CKD.
Risk Factor: Individuals with these systemic diseases may have an elevated risk of kidney complications.

8. Aging:

Cause: Aging itself can result in gradual changes in kidney structure and function, making older individuals more susceptible to CKD.
Risk Factor: Advancing age is considered a risk factor for the development of CKD.

9. Cardiovascular Disease:

Cause: Cardiovascular conditions, including heart failure and atherosclerosis, can impact kidney function by affecting blood flow to the kidneys.
Risk Factor: Individuals with existing cardiovascular diseases may have an increased risk of CKD.

10. Smoking and Substance Abuse:

Cause: Smoking and certain substance abuses, such as excessive alcohol consumption or illicit drug use, can contribute to kidney damage.
Risk Factor: Individuals engaging in these behaviors may be at a higher risk of CKD.

11. Genetic Factors:

Cause: Some individuals may have an inherited predisposition to kidney disease due to specific genetic factors.
Risk Factor: Family history of kidney disease may increase the risk for certain individuals.

12. Obesity:

Cause: Obesity is associated with an increased risk of diabetes and hypertension, both of which are major causes of CKD.
Risk Factor: Individuals with obesity may be at a higher risk of developing CKD.

Stages of Chronic Kidney Disease

Chronic Kidney Disease (CKD) is classified into five stages, each indicating the level of kidney function and the severity of damage. The staging system is based on the estimated Glomerular Filtration Rate (eGFR), which is a measure of how well the kidneys are filtering waste from the blood. The stages range from Stage 1, representing mild kidney damage, to Stage 5, indicating end-stage renal disease (ESRD). Here's an in-depth look at each stage:

Stage 1: Kidney Damage with Normal or High eGFR ($\geq$90 mL/min/1.73m^2)

Description: In this early stage, kidney damage is present, but the eGFR is still normal or even higher than average.

Clinical Features: Patients may not experience noticeable symptoms, and the condition may be detected through routine blood or urine tests.

Management: Focus is on identifying and managing underlying causes, such as hypertension or diabetes, and implementing lifestyle changes to slow progression.

Stage 2: Kidney Damage with Mildly Reduced eGFR (60-89 mL/min/1.73m²)

Description: Kidney damage is still present, and there is a mild reduction in the eGFR.

Clinical Features: Similar to Stage 1, symptoms may be minimal, and early detection is often through routine screening.

Management: Emphasis on lifestyle modifications, blood pressure control, and addressing underlying conditions to prevent further decline.

Stage 3: Moderate Reduction in eGFR (30-59 mL/min/1.73m²)

Description: Kidney function is moderately reduced, indicating a more advanced stage of CKD.

Clinical Features: Patients may begin to experience symptoms such as fatigue, fluid retention, and changes in urination.

Management: Comprehensive management includes dietary adjustments, blood pressure control, and monitoring for complications. Referral to a nephrologist may be considered.

Stage 4: Severe Reduction in eGFR (15-29 mL/min/1.73m²)

Description: Kidney function is significantly reduced, and patients are at higher risk of complications.
Clinical Features: Symptoms become more pronounced, including anemia, bone disorders, and increased susceptibility to infections.
Management: Intensive management to slow progression, along with potential preparation for renal replacement therapy (dialysis or transplantation). Consultation with a nephrologist is essential.

Stage 5: End-Stage Renal Disease (ESRD) (eGFR <15 mL/min/1.73m² or on Dialysis)

Description: Kidney function is severely impaired, and patients may require renal replacement therapy for survival.
Clinical Features: Symptoms are pronounced, and patients may experience fatigue, nausea, itching, and other complications.
Management: Options include dialysis (hemodialysis or peritoneal dialysis) or kidney transplantation. End-of-life care considerations may also be discussed.

Notes:

The progression from one stage to the next is not uniform, and individuals may remain in a particular stage for an extended period.

Regular monitoring, lifestyle modifications, and management of underlying conditions are crucial to slowing the progression of CKD.

Early detection and intervention, especially in the earlier stages, can significantly impact the course of the disease and improve outcomes.

PART 2

Making Smart Food Choices for Kidney Health

Embracing Whole and Minimally Processed Foods

Nutrition plays a pivotal role in the management of chronic kidney disease (CKD), influencing overall health and well-being. Embracing a diet rich in whole and minimally processed foods can be particularly beneficial for individuals with kidney disease, as it helps control key nutritional components while reducing the intake of substances that may be harmful to compromised kidneys. Here's a detailed exploration of the principles and benefits of incorporating whole and minimally processed foods into a kidney-friendly diet:

1. Fresh Fruits and Vegetables:

Benefits: Rich in vitamins, minerals, and antioxidants, fruits and vegetables provide essential nutrients without contributing excessive amounts of sodium, potassium, or phosphorus. Choose varieties with lower potassium content, such as apples, berries, and green beans.

2. Lean Proteins:

Benefits: Incorporating lean protein sources, such as poultry, fish, and eggs, can help meet protein needs without overloading the kidneys with excess waste products. Moderation is key, and portion control is essential to avoid excessive protein intake.

3. Whole Grains:

Benefits: Whole grains like brown rice, quinoa, and whole wheat products provide fiber, B-vitamins, and energy without contributing significantly to potassium and phosphorus levels. These grains promote digestive health and help regulate blood sugar.

4. Healthy Fats:

Benefits: Opt for heart-healthy fats from sources like olive oil, avocados, and nuts. These fats support overall health and provide a good source of calories without negatively impacting kidney function.

5. Limited Sodium Intake:

Benefits: Minimizing sodium (salt) is crucial to managing blood pressure and fluid balance. Choose fresh, unprocessed foods, and use herbs and spices for flavoring instead of salt. Be mindful of hidden sources of sodium in processed foods.

6. Controlled Potassium Intake:

Benefits: While fruits and vegetables are essential, monitoring potassium intake is crucial for individuals with kidney disease. Opt for lower-potassium options and control portions to maintain a balance that supports kidney health.

7. Phosphorus Management:

Benefits: Whole foods, particularly those low in phosphorus, can help manage phosphorus levels. Choose dairy alternatives, grains, and lean proteins with lower phosphorus content. Limiting processed and fast foods can help control phosphorus intake.

8. Hydration with Water:

Benefits: Staying adequately hydrated with water is vital for kidney function. It helps flush out toxins and aids in maintaining a proper fluid balance. Limiting sugary beverages and excessive caffeine is advisable.

9. Monitoring Calcium Intake:

Benefits: While calcium is important for bone health, excessive intake can contribute to complications in kidney disease. Choose moderate amounts of dairy or dairy alternatives and be mindful of calcium supplements.

10. Individualized Approach:

Benefits: Every individual with kidney disease is unique, and dietary recommendations should be tailored to individual needs, including stage of CKD, comorbid conditions, and personal preferences. Consultation with a registered dietitian or healthcare professional is essential to create a personalized nutrition plan.

11. Reading Food Labels:

Benefits: Be vigilant in reading food labels to identify hidden sources of sodium, potassium, and phosphorus in packaged foods. Opt for products with minimal additives and processing.

A Guide to Kidney-Friendly Whole Foods and their Benefits

Adopting a kidney-friendly diet involves making mindful choices about the types of foods consumed to support optimal kidney function and overall well-being. Here's a comprehensive guide to kidney-friendly whole foods, along with their benefits:

1. Low-Potassium Fruits:

Examples: Apples, berries, grapes, and watermelon.
Benefits: Low-potassium fruits are rich in vitamins, antioxidants, and fiber without contributing excess potassium. They provide essential nutrients without overloading the kidneys.

2. Cruciferous Vegetables:

Examples: Cauliflower, cabbage, and broccoli.
Benefits: These vegetables are low in potassium and phosphorus, making them suitable choices for kidney health. They also offer fiber and various vitamins.

3. Berries:

Examples: Blueberries, strawberries, and raspberries.
Benefits: Berries are low in potassium and high in antioxidants, which help combat inflammation. They provide a flavorful addition to meals and snacks without overloading on nutrients that may stress the kidneys.

4. Red Bell Peppers:

Benefits: Red bell peppers are a low-potassium vegetable rich in vitamins A, C, and B6. They add color and flavor to dishes while providing essential nutrients.

5. Egg Whites:

Benefits: Egg whites are a high-quality protein source with low phosphorus content. They provide amino acids without contributing to excessive waste product buildup in the kidneys.

6. Skinless Poultry:

Examples: Chicken and turkey.
Benefits: Lean, skinless poultry is a protein source that is lower in phosphorus and potassium compared to red meats. It supports muscle health without placing additional strain on the kidneys.

7. Fish:

Examples: Salmon, trout, and tuna (in moderation).
Benefits: Fatty fish like salmon provide omega-3 fatty acids, which have anti-inflammatory properties. Fish is a good protein source with lower phosphorus content compared to some other meats.

8. Olive Oil:

Benefits: Olive oil is a heart-healthy fat that can be used in cooking and salad dressings. It provides monounsaturated fats without contributing to excessive sodium levels.

9. Cauliflower:

Benefits: Cauliflower is a versatile and low-potassium vegetable that can be used as a substitute for higher-potassium foods. It's an excellent source of fiber, vitamin C, and folate.

10. Garlic:

Benefits: Garlic adds flavor to dishes without contributing to sodium levels. It has anti-inflammatory properties and may have potential cardiovascular benefits.

11. Cabbage:

Benefits: Cabbage is a low-potassium and low-phosphorus vegetable. It provides fiber, vitamins, and antioxidants while supporting a kidney-friendly diet.

12. Pineapple:

Benefits: Pineapple is a tropical fruit with lower potassium content. It provides vitamin C, manganese, and digestive enzymes, making it a refreshing and kidney-friendly choice.

13. Quinoa:

Benefits: Quinoa is a whole grain that offers a good source of protein, fiber, and various vitamins and minerals. It is lower in phosphorus compared to some other grains.

14. Cauliflower Rice:

Benefits: Cauliflower rice is a low-carbohydrate and low-potassium alternative to traditional rice. It can be a versatile base for various dishes.

15. Red Grapes:

Benefits: Red grapes are a kidney-friendly fruit rich in antioxidants, including resveratrol. They provide natural sweetness without contributing excessive potassium.

16. Limited Portion Control:

Benefits: Practicing portion control is essential for managing nutrient intake. It helps prevent excessive consumption of nutrients like potassium and phosphorus while still enjoying a variety of foods.

17. Hydration with Water:

Benefits: Staying hydrated with water is crucial for kidney function. It aids in flushing out toxins and maintaining proper fluid balance without contributing to nutrient overload.

18. Low-Sodium Herbs and Spices:

Benefits: Using herbs and spices for flavoring instead of salt helps control sodium intake. This promotes a kidney-friendly diet while enhancing the taste of meals.

19. Cucumber:

Benefits: Cucumbers are a hydrating, low-potassium vegetable that adds crunch to salads and snacks. They are a refreshing choice with minimal impact on nutrient levels.

20. Cranberries:

Benefits: Cranberries are low in potassium and can be incorporated into the diet as juice or sauce. They offer potential benefits for urinary tract health.

Eating Low-Glycemic and Anti-Inflammatory Foods

Adopting a diet rich in low-glycemic and anti-inflammatory foods is recognized as a proactive approach to promoting overall health and well-being. These dietary principles are particularly beneficial for managing conditions such as diabetes, metabolic syndrome, and chronic inflammatory disorders. Here's a detailed exploration of the concepts behind low-glycemic and anti-inflammatory eating, along with examples of foods that align with these principles:

Low-Glycemic Eating:

1. Understanding the Glycemic Index (GI):

- Definition: The glycemic index measures how quickly a carbohydrate-containing food raises blood sugar levels. Foods are categorized as low, medium, or high glycemic based on this scale.
- Benefits: Choosing low-glycemic foods helps regulate blood sugar levels, promoting more stable energy levels and reducing the risk of insulin resistance and type 2 diabetes.

2. Examples of Low-Glycemic Foods:

- Non-Starchy Vegetables: Leafy greens, broccoli, cauliflower, peppers.
- Legumes: Lentils, chickpeas, black beans.
- Whole Grains: Quinoa, barley, bulgur, and whole wheat products.

- Nuts and Seeds: Almonds, walnuts, chia seeds.
- Dairy: Greek yogurt, cottage cheese.
- Fruits: Berries, cherries, apples, and pears.

3. Benefits of Low-Glycemic Eating:

- Stable Blood Sugar: Low-glycemic foods release glucose slowly, preventing rapid spikes and crashes in blood sugar levels.
- Improved Satiety: These foods often contribute to a feeling of fullness, helping with weight management.
- Reduced Risk of Type 2 Diabetes: A low-glycemic diet may lower the risk of developing insulin resistance and type 2 diabetes.

Anti-Inflammatory Eating:

1. Understanding Inflammation:

- Definition: Inflammation is the body's natural response to injury or infection. However, chronic inflammation is associated with various health conditions, including cardiovascular disease, arthritis, and certain autoimmune disorders.
- Benefits: Anti-inflammatory eating focuses on reducing chronic inflammation to support overall health and lower the risk of inflammatory-related diseases.

2. Examples of Anti-Inflammatory Foods:

- Fatty Fish: Salmon, mackerel, and sardines rich in omega-3 fatty acids.
- Leafy Greens: Kale, spinach, and Swiss chard.
- Berries: Blueberries, strawberries, and raspberries.
- Turmeric and Ginger: Spices with anti-inflammatory compounds.
- Nuts and Seeds: Walnuts, flaxseeds, and chia seeds.
- Olive Oil: Extra virgin olive oil with anti-inflammatory properties.
- Colorful Fruits and Vegetables: Tomatoes, peppers, and oranges with diverse antioxidants.

3. Benefits of Anti-Inflammatory Eating:

- Reduced Chronic Disease Risk: Anti-inflammatory foods may lower the risk of chronic diseases, including cardiovascular disease and certain cancers.
- Improved Joint Health: Anti-inflammatory eating can benefit individuals with inflammatory joint conditions like arthritis.
- Enhanced Immune Function: A diet rich in anti-inflammatory foods supports a robust immune system.

Integrating Both Principles:

1. Whole, Unprocessed Foods:
Choosing whole, unprocessed foods naturally aligns with both low-glycemic and anti-inflammatory principles. These foods are rich in nutrients, fiber, and antioxidants.

2. Balanced Macronutrients:
Including a balance of carbohydrates, proteins, and healthy fats in meals promotes stable blood sugar levels and provides essential nutrients.

3. Mindful Eating:
Being mindful of portion sizes and eating slowly allows for better regulation of blood sugar levels and may prevent overeating, supporting both low-glycemic and anti-inflammatory goals.

4. Hydration:
Staying well-hydrated with water and incorporating herbal teas supports overall health and can contribute to an anti-inflammatory lifestyle.

5. Individualized Approach:
Recognizing that individual responses to foods may vary, an individualized approach to low-glycemic and anti-inflammatory eating is crucial. Factors such as genetics, existing health conditions, and lifestyle should be considered.

Minimizing High-Glycemic and Inflammatory Foods

Dietary choices play a significant role in overall health, and certain foods can contribute to conditions like inflammation and disruptions in blood sugar levels.

Minimizing the intake of high-glycemic and inflammatory foods is a proactive approach to support general well-being and may be particularly beneficial for individuals managing conditions like diabetes, metabolic syndrome, or chronic inflammatory disorders. Here's a detailed exploration of strategies to minimize high-glycemic and inflammatory foods:

1. Understanding the Glycemic Index (GI):

- Definition: The Glycemic Index is a scale that ranks carbohydrate-containing foods based on how quickly they raise blood sugar levels.
- Strategy: Choose low-GI foods to help stabilize blood sugar levels, preventing rapid spikes and crashes.

2. Limiting Refined Carbohydrates:
- Examples: White bread, white rice, sugary cereals, and pastries.
- Strategy: Opt for whole grains like brown rice, quinoa, and whole wheat, which have a lower GI and provide more sustained energy.

3. Choosing Whole, Unprocessed Foods:
   - Examples: Fresh fruits, vegetables, lean proteins, and whole grains.
   - Strategy: Whole foods are generally lower on the glycemic index and offer a range of essential nutrients, promoting overall health and reducing the risk of inflammation.

4. Incorporating Fiber-Rich Foods:
   - Examples: Legumes, vegetables, fruits, and whole grains.
   - Strategy: Fiber slows down the digestion and absorption of carbohydrates, helping to regulate blood sugar levels and promote a feeling of fullness.

5. Balancing Macronutrients:
   - Strategy: Include a balance of carbohydrates, proteins, and healthy fats in each meal. This combination can help stabilize blood sugar levels and provide sustained energy.

6. Avoiding Sugary Beverages:
   - Examples: Soda, fruit juices, and energy drinks.
   - Strategy: Opt for water, herbal teas, or unsweetened alternatives to minimize added sugars and prevent spikes in blood sugar.

7. Monitoring Portion Sizes:
   - Strategy: Be mindful of portion sizes to avoid overconsumption of high-glycemic foods. This practice helps regulate calorie intake and maintains steady blood sugar levels.

8. Reducing Processed Foods:
   - Examples: Processed snacks, fast food, and packaged meals.
   - Strategy: Processed foods often contain added sugars and unhealthy fats. Choosing whole, minimally processed options can help minimize the inflammatory impact of these ingredients.

9. Opting for Healthy Fats:
   - Examples: Avocados, olive oil, nuts, and fatty fish.
   - Strategy: Healthy fats have anti-inflammatory properties. Including them in the diet can help balance blood sugar levels and support overall health.

10. Identifying and Avoiding Food Sensitivities:
   - Strategy: Some individuals may have specific food sensitivities that contribute to inflammation. Identifying and eliminating trigger foods can help manage inflammatory responses.

11. Including Anti-Inflammatory Spices:
   - Examples: Turmeric, ginger, garlic, and cinnamon.
   - Strategy: These spices contain compounds with anti-inflammatory properties. Incorporating them into meals not only adds flavor but also provides potential health benefits.

12. Choosing Low-Glycemic Sweeteners:
   - Examples: Stevia, monk fruit, and erythritol.
   - Strategy: When a sweetener is needed, opt for those with a lower impact on blood sugar to avoid spikes.

13. Managing Stress:
   - Strategy: Chronic stress can contribute to inflammation and impact blood sugar levels. Adopt stress-management techniques such as mindfulness, meditation, or exercise.

14. Seeking Professional Guidance:
   - Strategy: Consult with healthcare professionals, including dietitians or nutritionists, to create a personalized plan that aligns with individual health goals and dietary needs.

Minimizing high-glycemic and inflammatory foods involves making informed and intentional choices about dietary habits. This approach not only supports conditions like diabetes and inflammatory disorders but also promotes overall health and well-being.

Part 3

Managing Diabetes and Kidney Health Together

Demystifying the Glycemic Index

Individuals managing both diabetes and kidney health face unique challenges in maintaining stable blood sugar levels while also supporting optimal kidney function. The glycemic index (GI) is a valuable tool that can be particularly beneficial in navigating these dual health concerns. Here's an in-depth exploration of how understanding the glycemic index can contribute to the management of diabetes and kidney health concurrently:

1. Understanding the Glycemic Index:

Definition: The glycemic index is a numerical scale that ranks carbohydrates based on their impact on blood glucose levels. Foods with a high GI lead to a rapid spike in blood sugar, while those with a low GI result in a slower, more gradual increase.

Importance for Diabetes: For individuals with diabetes, managing blood sugar levels is crucial to prevent hyperglycemia (high blood sugar) and its associated complications.

2. Benefits for Managing Blood Sugar in Diabetes:

Low-GI Foods: Choosing low-GI carbohydrates can help regulate blood sugar levels, preventing sudden spikes and crashes. This is especially important for individuals with diabetes, as stable blood sugar is key to long-term health.

Sustained Energy: Low-GI foods provide a sustained release of energy, promoting stable blood sugar throughout the day. This can help manage energy levels and reduce the risk of hypoglycemia (low blood sugar).

3. Relevance to Kidney Health:

Phosphorus Consideration: Some high-GI foods may be rich in phosphorus, which is a concern for individuals with compromised kidney function. A diet with a balanced GI can help manage phosphorus intake.

Blood Pressure Control: The GI is linked to blood pressure regulation. Maintaining blood pressure within a healthy range is crucial for kidney health, especially in individuals with diabetes who may be at an increased risk of kidney complications.

4. Key Considerations for Diabetes and Kidney Health:

Low-GI Foods: Prioritize low-GI foods such as whole grains, legumes, non-starchy vegetables, and certain fruits to manage blood sugar levels without putting excess strain on the kidneys.

Protein Choices: Opt for lean protein sources, as high-protein diets can sometimes be associated with increased kidney workload. Incorporate plant-based proteins, fish, and poultry while monitoring portion sizes.

Limiting Processed Foods: Highly processed and sugary foods often have a high GI and may also contribute to an increased risk of kidney damage. Limiting the intake of these foods is beneficial for both diabetes and kidney health.

5. Practical Tips for Managing Diabetes and Kidney Health:

Meal Planning: Incorporate a variety of low-GI foods into meals to promote blood sugar control and support kidney health.

Balanced Meals: Combine low-GI carbohydrates with lean proteins, healthy fats, and fiber-rich foods to create balanced meals that benefit both diabetes and kidney function.

Hydration: Staying well-hydrated is crucial for kidney health. Water is the best choice, and individuals with diabetes should be mindful of sugar content in beverages.

Regular Monitoring: Regularly monitor blood sugar levels, kidney function (through tests like estimated glomerular filtration rate or eGFR), and other relevant health indicators. This helps in making informed adjustments to the diet and lifestyle.

6. Potential Challenges:

Individual Variability: Responses to the same food can vary among individuals. It's essential to consider personal factors and consult with healthcare professionals for personalized guidance.

Phosphorus Awareness: While the GI is a valuable tool, it does not specifically address phosphorus content. Individuals with kidney concerns should also be mindful of phosphorus-rich foods.

7. Consultation with Healthcare Professionals:

Collaborating with a registered dietitian, endocrinologist, and nephrologist is crucial for individuals managing both diabetes and kidney health. They can provide personalized guidance, consider individual health needs, and offer comprehensive support.

Demystifying the glycemic index in the context of managing diabetes and kidney health together involves making informed and intentional food choices. By understanding the impact of carbohydrates on blood sugar and considering the potential implications for kidney health, individuals can create a balanced and nourishing diet that addresses both aspects of their health.

The Power of a Low-Glycemic Diet for Your Health

A low-glycemic diet has emerged as a powerful tool for promoting overall health and well-being, particularly in the management of conditions like diabetes, obesity, heart disease, and even kidney disease. This dietary approach focuses on consuming foods that have a minimal impact on blood sugar levels, which can have numerous benefits for various aspects of health. Here's an in-depth exploration of the power of a low-glycemic diet and its impact on health:

1. Blood Sugar Control:

Stabilized Blood Glucose Levels: Low-glycemic foods are digested and absorbed more slowly, resulting in gradual increases in blood sugar levels. This prevents spikes and crashes in blood glucose, promoting more stable energy levels throughout the day.

Reduced Risk of Diabetes: By avoiding rapid fluctuations in blood sugar, a low-glycemic diet can help prevent the onset of type 2 diabetes and improve glycemic control in individuals with diabetes.

2. Weight Management:

Increased Satiety: Low-glycemic foods tend to be rich in fiber and protein, which promote feelings of fullness and satiety. This can help control appetite and reduce overall calorie intake, supporting weight loss efforts.

Reduced Fat Storage: High-glycemic foods can lead to excess insulin secretion, which promotes fat storage. By choosing low-glycemic options, individuals may be less prone to weight gain and obesity-related health issues.

3. Heart Health:

Improved Lipid Profile: Low-glycemic foods have been associated with improvements in cholesterol levels, including reductions in LDL (bad) cholesterol and triglycerides, and increases in HDL (good) cholesterol, which can lower the risk of heart disease.

Lower Blood Pressure: The gradual release of glucose from low-glycemic foods helps prevent sudden spikes in insulin, which may contribute to improved blood pressure control and reduced risk of hypertension.

4. Reduced Inflammation:

Anti-Inflammatory Effects: High-glycemic foods can trigger inflammatory responses in the body, whereas low-glycemic foods have been shown to have anti-inflammatory properties. This can help reduce the risk of chronic inflammation and associated diseases.

Protection Against Chronic Diseases: Chronic inflammation is linked to the development of various diseases, including heart disease, cancer, and autoimmune conditions. By reducing inflammation, a low-glycemic diet may help protect against these conditions.

5. Enhanced Energy Levels:

Steady Energy Release: Low-glycemic foods provide a sustained release of energy, helping to prevent energy crashes and fatigue commonly associated with high-glycemic meals.

Improved Mental Focus: Stable blood sugar levels support cognitive function and mental clarity, allowing for better focus and concentration throughout the day.

6. Kidney Health:

Supports Kidney Function: For individuals with kidney disease, maintaining stable blood sugar levels is essential for preserving kidney function and preventing further damage. A low-glycemic diet helps achieve this goal by avoiding sudden spikes in blood glucose.

Reduces Risk of Complications: High blood sugar levels can exacerbate kidney damage in individuals with diabetes or kidney disease. By following a low-glycemic diet, individuals can reduce their risk of complications and slow the progression of kidney disease.

7. Practical Tips for Following a Low-Glycemic Diet:

Focus on Whole Foods: Choose whole, minimally processed foods such as fruits, vegetables, whole grains, lean proteins, and healthy fats.

Read Food Labels: Pay attention to the glycemic index and glycemic load of foods when grocery shopping. Opt for low-glycemic options whenever possible.

Balance Meals: Include a combination of carbohydrates, protein, and healthy fats in each meal to slow down digestion and stabilize blood sugar levels.

Monitor Portion Sizes: Even low-glycemic foods can contribute to elevated blood sugar levels if consumed in large quantities. Practice portion control to maintain balance.

Making a Low-Glycemic Lifestyle Work for You

Transitioning to a low-glycemic lifestyle involves more than just choosing low-glycemic foods—it requires adopting sustainable habits and making practical changes to your daily routine. Whether you're managing diabetes, aiming for weight loss, or simply prioritizing your overall health, here's a detailed guide on how to make a low-glycemic lifestyle work for you:

1. Educate Yourself:

Understand Glycemic Index (GI): Learn about the GI and how different foods affect blood sugar levels. Familiarize yourself with the GI values of common foods and ingredients.

Glycemic Load (GL): Consider both the GI and portion sizes when assessing the impact of foods on blood sugar levels. Lowering the GL of meals can further support stable blood glucose control.

2. Plan Your Meals:

Create Balanced Meals: Design meals that incorporate a variety of low-glycemic carbohydrates, lean proteins, healthy fats, and fiber-rich foods.

Meal Prepping: Plan and prepare meals and snacks ahead of time to ensure you have nutritious options readily available. This reduces the temptation to reach for high-glycemic convenience foods.

3. Choose Low-Glycemic Foods:

Whole Foods: Prioritize whole, unprocessed foods such as fruits, vegetables, legumes, whole grains, lean proteins, and nuts/seeds.

Fiber-Rich Options: Include plenty of fiber-rich foods like beans, lentils, oats, and vegetables, as fiber helps slow down the digestion and absorption of carbohydrates, resulting in a lower glycemic response.

4. Be Mindful of Portions:

Portion Control: Practice mindful eating and be aware of portion sizes. Even low-glycemic foods can impact blood sugar levels if consumed in large quantities.

Use Smaller Plates: Opt for smaller plates and bowls to help control portion sizes and prevent overeating.

5. Incorporate Healthy Cooking Methods:

Grilling, Steaming, and Baking: Use cooking methods that require minimal added fats and oils to keep meals lower in calories and saturated fats.

Limit Added Sugars: Avoid excessive use of sweeteners and added sugars in cooking and baking, as they can increase the glycemic load of meals.

6. Practice Snacking Wisely:

Choose Nutrient-Dense Snacks: Opt for low-glycemic snacks such as fresh fruit, raw vegetables with hummus, Greek yogurt, nuts/seeds, or whole-grain crackers with cheese.

Portion-Controlled Snacks: Pre-portion snacks into single servings to avoid mindless eating and help manage blood sugar levels.

7. Stay Hydrated:

Drink Plenty of Water: Stay hydrated by drinking water throughout the day. Thirst can sometimes be mistaken for hunger, leading to unnecessary snacking.
8. Monitor Your Progress:

Keep Track of Your Meals: Use a food journal or mobile app to record your meals, snacks, and portion sizes. This can help you identify patterns and make adjustments as needed.

Track Blood Sugar Levels: If you have diabetes, monitor your blood glucose levels regularly to assess the impact of your dietary choices on glycemic control.

9. Practice Flexibility and Moderation:

Allow for Treats Occasionally: It's okay to enjoy occasional indulgences, but be mindful of portion sizes and frequency. Incorporating treats into your overall dietary pattern in moderation can help you maintain a sustainable low-glycemic lifestyle.

Focus on Progress, Not Perfection: Aim for consistency rather than perfection. Making gradual changes and focusing on long-term habits is key to sustaining a low-glycemic lifestyle.

10. Seek Support and Guidance:

Consult a Registered Dietitian: Work with a registered dietitian or healthcare professional who can provide personalized guidance and support for incorporating a low-glycemic lifestyle into your routine.

Join Support Groups: Consider joining support groups or online communities where you can connect with others who are following a similar dietary approach and share tips and experiences.

Part 4:

The Essential Potassium, Phosphorus, and Sodium Counter

Baked Goods

Whole Wheat Bread:
Potassium: 80mg
Phosphorus: 40mg
Sodium: 150mg

Banana Bread:
Potassium: 150mg
Phosphorus: 60mg
Sodium: 200mg

Blueberry Muffins:
Potassium: 120mg
Phosphorus: 50mg
Sodium: 180mg

Apple Pie:
Potassium: 150mg
Phosphorus: 60mg
Sodium: 200mg

Chocolate Chip Cookies:
Potassium: 60mg
Phosphorus: 40mg
Sodium: 100mg

Lemon Bars:
Potassium: 80mg
Phosphorus: 30mg
Sodium: 120mg

Pumpkin Bread:
Potassium: 120mg
Phosphorus: 50mg
Sodium: 180mg

Cinnamon Rolls:
Potassium: 100mg
Phosphorus: 60mg
Sodium: 150mg

Zucchini Bread:
Potassium: 150mg
Phosphorus: 50mg
Sodium: 200mg

Cranberry Scones:
Potassium: 90mg
Phosphorus: 40mg
Sodium: 150mg

Chocolate Brownies:
Potassium: 70mg
Phosphorus: 50mg
Sodium: 120mg

Raspberry Danish:
Potassium: 100mg
Phosphorus: 60mg

     THE COMPLETE FOODS LISTS FOR KIDNEY DISEAS

Sodium: 180mg

Oatmeal Raisin Cookies:
Potassium: 80mg
Phosphorus: 40mg
Sodium: 120mg

Carrot Cake:
Potassium: 120mg
Phosphorus: 70mg
Sodium: 180mg

Almond Biscotti:
Potassium: 60mg
Phosphorus: 40mg
Sodium: 100mg

Peanut Butter Cookies:
Potassium: 70mg
Phosphorus: 50mg
Sodium: 120mg

Chocolate Cake:
Potassium: 130mg
Phosphorus: 80mg
Sodium: 200mg

Cherry Pie:
Potassium: 140mg
Phosphorus: 70mg
Sodium: 180mg

Angel Food Cake:
Potassium: 70mg
Phosphorus: 30mg
Sodium: 100mg

Pecan Pie:
Potassium: 160mg
Phosphorus: 90mg
Sodium: 200mg

Date Bars:
Potassium: 90mg
Phosphorus: 50mg
Sodium: 150mg

Shortbread Cookies:
Potassium: 50mg
Phosphorus: 40mg
Sodium: 100mg

Coffee Cake:
Potassium: 110mg
Phosphorus: 60mg
Sodium: 150mg

Fig Newtons:
Potassium: 100mg
Phosphorus: 40mg
Sodium: 120mg

Marble Cake:
Potassium: 140mg
Phosphorus: 70mg

Sodium: 180mg

Pineapple Upside-Down Cake:
Potassium: 120mg
Phosphorus: 60mg
Sodium: 160mg

Cinnamon Swirl Bread:
Potassium: 110mg
Phosphorus: 50mg
Sodium: 140mg

Gingerbread Cookies:
Potassium: 60mg
Phosphorus: 40mg
Sodium: 110mg

Pita Bread:
Potassium: 50mg
Phosphorus: 40mg
Sodium: 150mg

Bagels:
Potassium: 60mg
Phosphorus: 50mg
Sodium: 200mg

Cornbread:
Potassium: 80mg
Phosphorus: 40mg
Sodium: 170mg

Irish Soda Bread:
Potassium: 70mg
Phosphorus: 40mg
Sodium: 140mg

Rye Bread:
Potassium: 60mg
Phosphorus: 40mg
Sodium: 160mg

French Baguette:
Potassium: 60mg
Phosphorus: 40mg
Sodium: 200mg

Croissants:
Potassium: 80mg
Phosphorus: 50mg
Sodium: 210mg

Dinner Rolls:
Potassium: 60mg
Phosphorus: 40mg
Sodium: 180mg

Focaccia Bread:
Potassium: 70mg
Phosphorus: 50mg
Sodium: 190mg

Biscuits:
Potassium: 50mg
Phosphorus: 40mg

Sodium: 180mg

Cinnamon Raisin Bread:
Potassium: 90mg
Phosphorus: 50mg
Sodium: 180mg

Challah Bread:
Potassium: 60mg
Phosphorus: 40mg
Sodium: 180mg

Beans, Lentils, and Kidney-Friendly Choices

Black Beans:
Potassium: 230mg
Phosphorus: 45mg
Sodium: 1mg

Chickpeas (Garbanzo Beans):
Potassium: 210mg
Phosphorus: 70mg
Sodium: 10mg

Kidney Beans:
Potassium: 215mg
Phosphorus: 45mg
Sodium: 1mg

Lentils:
Potassium: 230mg
Phosphorus: 50mg
Sodium: 1mg

Navy Beans:
Potassium: 200mg
Phosphorus: 45mg
Sodium: 1mg

Pinto Beans:
Potassium: 220mg
Phosphorus: 45mg
Sodium: 1mg

Black-eyed Peas:
Potassium: 240mg
Phosphorus: 45mg
Sodium: 1mg

Split Peas:
Potassium: 200mg
Phosphorus: 65mg
Sodium: 1mg

Adzuki Beans:
Potassium: 200mg
Phosphorus: 55mg
Sodium: 1mg

Soybeans (Edamame):
Potassium: 180mg
Phosphorus: 90mg
Sodium: 1mg

Mung Beans:
Potassium: 210mg
Phosphorus: 50mg

Sodium: 1mg

Lima Beans:
Potassium: 215mg
Phosphorus: 45mg
Sodium: 1mg

Great Northern Beans:
Potassium: 220mg
Phosphorus: 45mg
Sodium: 1mg

Cannellini Beans:
Potassium: 200mg
Phosphorus: 45mg
Sodium: 1mg

Green Lentils:
Potassium: 230mg
Phosphorus: 50mg
Sodium: 1mg

Red Lentils:
Potassium: 240mg
Phosphorus: 50mg
Sodium: 1mg

Yellow Lentils:
Potassium: 230mg
Phosphorus: 50mg
Sodium: 1mg

French Green Lentils:
Potassium: 220mg
Phosphorus: 45mg
Sodium: 1mg

Black Lentils (Beluga Lentils):
Potassium: 230mg
Phosphorus: 50mg
Sodium: 1mg

Cranberry Beans:
Potassium: 210mg
Phosphorus: 45mg
Sodium: 1mg

Chickpea Flour (Besan):
Potassium: 280mg
Phosphorus: 150mg
Sodium: 10mg

Lentil Flour:
Potassium: 230mg
Phosphorus: 100mg
Sodium: 5mg

Black Bean Flour:
Potassium: 240mg
Phosphorus: 120mg
Sodium: 10mg

Soy Flour:
Potassium: 660mg
Phosphorus: 680mg

Sodium: 13mg

Red Kidney Bean Flour:
Potassium: 250mg
Phosphorus: 140mg
Sodium: 2mg

Yellow Split Peas:
Potassium: 200mg
Phosphorus: 60mg
Sodium: 1mg

Black Bean Pasta:
Potassium: 230mg
Phosphorus: 60mg
Sodium: 5mg

Chickpea Pasta:
Potassium: 200mg
Phosphorus: 65mg
Sodium: 5mg

Lentil Pasta:
Potassium: 240mg
Phosphorus: 70mg
Sodium: 5mg

Soy Milk:
Potassium: 90mg
Phosphorus: 80mg
Sodium: 100mg

Tofu:
Potassium: 120mg
Phosphorus: 150mg
Sodium: 5mg

Tempeh:
Potassium: 300mg
Phosphorus: 200mg
Sodium: 15mg

Black Bean Soup:
Potassium: 300mg
Phosphorus: 80mg
Sodium: 600mg

Lentil Soup:
Potassium: 350mg
Phosphorus: 120mg
Sodium: 600mg

Minestrone Soup:
Potassium: 350mg
Phosphorus: 120mg
Sodium: 650mg

Hummus:
Potassium: 220mg
Phosphorus: 80mg
Sodium: 180mg

Black Bean Salad:
Potassium: 280mg
Phosphorus: 100mg

     THE COMPLETE FOODS LISTS FOR KIDNEY DISEAS

Sodium: 200mg

Lentil Salad:
Potassium: 300mg
Phosphorus: 110mg
Sodium: 200mg

Three Bean Salad:
Potassium: 250mg
Phosphorus: 90mg
Sodium: 180mg

Bean Burritos:
Potassium: 320mg
Phosphorus: 120mg
Sodium: 300mg

Lentil Curry:
Potassium: 350mg
Phosphorus: 130mg
Sodium: 400mg

Black Bean Tacos:
Potassium: 310mg
Phosphorus: 100mg
Sodium: 250mg

Chickpea Salad:
Potassium: 280mg
Phosphorus: 100mg
Sodium: 200mg

Lentil Burgers:
Potassium: 330mg
Phosphorus: 120mg
Sodium: 300mg

Black Bean Chili:
Potassium: 350mg
Phosphorus: 110mg
Sodium: 400mg

Lentil Stew:
Potassium: 320mg
Phosphorus: 130mg
Sodium: 350mg

Chickpea Hummus Wrap:
Potassium: 320mg
Phosphorus: 110mg
Sodium: 280mg

Black Bean Quesadillas:
Potassium: 280mg
Phosphorus: 100mg
Sodium: 250mg

Lentil Shepherd's Pie:
Potassium: 330mg
Phosphorus: 120mg
Sodium: 320mg

Bean and Vegetable Stir-fry:
Potassium: 310mg
Phosphorus: 110mg

Sodium: 300mg

Beverages

Water:
Potassium: 0mg
Phosphorus: 0mg
Sodium: 0mg

Black Coffee (8 oz):
Potassium: 116mg
Phosphorus: 4mg
Sodium: 7mg

Green Tea (8 oz):
Potassium: 25mg
Phosphorus: 4mg
Sodium: 1mg

Herbal Tea (8 oz):
Potassium: 0mg
Phosphorus: 0mg
Sodium: 0mg

Plain Black Tea (8 oz):
Potassium: 88mg
Phosphorus: 2mg
Sodium: 2mg

Sparkling Water (8 oz):
Potassium: 0mg
Phosphorus: 0mg
Sodium: 0mg

Coconut Water (8 oz):
Potassium: 470mg
Phosphorus: 48mg
Sodium: 252mg

Orange Juice (8 oz):
Potassium: 450mg
Phosphorus: 26mg
Sodium: 0mg

Apple Juice (8 oz):
Potassium: 250mg
Phosphorus: 15mg
Sodium: 5mg

Cranberry Juice (8 oz):
Potassium: 135mg
Phosphorus: 13mg
Sodium: 2mg

Grape Juice (8 oz):
Potassium: 280mg
Phosphorus: 28mg
Sodium: 5mg

Pineapple Juice (8 oz):
Potassium: 180mg
Phosphorus: 13mg
Sodium: 2mg

Tomato Juice (8 oz):
Potassium: 530mg
Phosphorus: 44mg

Sodium: 650mg

Lemonade (8 oz):
Potassium: 15mg
Phosphorus: 8mg
Sodium: 10mg

Limeade (8 oz):
Potassium: 40mg
Phosphorus: 8mg
Sodium: 10mg

Vegetable Juice (8 oz):
Potassium: 350mg
Phosphorus: 18mg
Sodium: 480mg

Carrot Juice (8 oz):
Potassium: 690mg
Phosphorus: 41mg
Sodium: 75mg

Beet Juice (8 oz):
Potassium: 600mg
Phosphorus: 27mg
Sodium: 140mg

Grapefruit Juice (8 oz):
Potassium: 350mg
Phosphorus: 28mg
Sodium: 0mg

Pear Juice (8 oz):
Potassium: 255mg
Phosphorus: 15mg
Sodium: 5mg

Watermelon Juice (8 oz):
Potassium: 320mg
Phosphorus: 15mg
Sodium: 5mg

Peach Juice (8 oz):
Potassium: 230mg
Phosphorus: 15mg
Sodium: 5mg

Apricot Juice (8 oz):
Potassium: 280mg
Phosphorus: 15mg
Sodium: 10mg

Prune Juice (8 oz):
Potassium: 530mg
Phosphorus: 30mg
Sodium: 5mg

Papaya Juice (8 oz):
Potassium: 470mg
Phosphorus: 20mg
Sodium: 5mg

Mango Juice (8 oz):
Potassium: 320mg
Phosphorus: 25mg

Sodium: 10mg

Guava Juice (8 oz):
Potassium: 600mg
Phosphorus: 28mg
Sodium: 10mg

Passion Fruit Juice (8 oz):
Potassium: 500mg
Phosphorus: 20mg
Sodium: 15mg

Kiwi Juice (8 oz):
Potassium: 530mg
Phosphorus: 24mg
Sodium: 10mg

Blueberry Juice (8 oz):
Potassium: 450mg
Phosphorus: 26mg
Sodium: 2mg

Cherry Juice (8 oz):
Potassium: 300mg
Phosphorus: 20mg
Sodium: 5mg

Aloe Vera Juice (8 oz):
Potassium: 35mg
Phosphorus: 5mg
Sodium: 30mg

Wheatgrass Juice (8 oz):
Potassium: 400mg
Phosphorus: 40mg
Sodium: 5mg

Barley Grass Juice (8 oz):
Potassium: 430mg
Phosphorus: 35mg
Sodium: 10mg

Spirulina Drink (8 oz):
Potassium: 1000mg
Phosphorus: 200mg
Sodium: 150mg

Almond Milk (8 oz):
Potassium: 180mg
Phosphorus: 20mg
Sodium: 160mg

Soy Milk (8 oz):
Potassium: 160mg
Phosphorus: 95mg
Sodium: 80mg

Rice Milk (8 oz):
Potassium: 10mg
Phosphorus: 30mg
Sodium: 90mg

Oat Milk (8 oz):
Potassium: 120mg
Phosphorus: 90mg

Sodium: 100mg

Hemp Milk (8 oz):
Potassium: 130mg
Phosphorus: 180mg
Sodium: 140mg

Cashew Milk (8 oz):
Potassium: 45mg
Phosphorus: 20mg
Sodium: 160mg

Macadamia Milk (8 oz):
Potassium: 30mg
Phosphorus: 15mg
Sodium: 0mg

Hazelnut Milk (8 oz):
Potassium: 50mg
Phosphorus: 20mg
Sodium: 150mg

Flax Milk (8 oz):
Potassium: 150mg
Phosphorus: 110mg
Sodium: 100mg

Quinoa Milk (8 oz):
Potassium: 120mg
Phosphorus: 90mg
Sodium: 100mg

Walnut Milk (8 oz):
Potassium: 35mg
Phosphorus: 20mg
Sodium: 80mg

Pistachio Milk (8 oz):
Potassium: 30mg
Phosphorus: 15mg
Sodium: 40mg

Brazil Nut Milk (8 oz):
Potassium: 90mg
Phosphorus: 30mg
Sodium: 5mg

Pea Milk (8 oz):
Potassium: 100mg
Phosphorus: 80mg
Sodium: 95mg

Potato Juice (8 oz):
Potassium: 1100mg
Phosphorus: 65mg
Sodium: 20mg

 THE COMPLETE FOODS LISTS FOR KIDNEY DISEAS

Cheerios:
Potassium: 115mg
Phosphorus: 70mg
Sodium: 160mg

Corn Flakes:
Potassium: 25mg
Phosphorus: 45mg
Sodium: 200mg

Rice Krispies:
Potassium: 20mg
Phosphorus: 30mg
Sodium: 130mg

Special K:
Potassium: 80mg
Phosphorus: 50mg
Sodium: 210mg

Raisin Bran:
Potassium: 260mg
Phosphorus: 110mg
Sodium: 340mg

Frosted Flakes:
Potassium: 40mg
Phosphorus: 50mg
Sodium: 150mg

Honey Nut Cheerios:
Potassium: 115mg

Phosphorus: 70mg
Sodium: 190mg

Froot Loops:
Potassium: 25mg
Phosphorus: 50mg
Sodium: 150mg

Cocoa Pebbles:
Potassium: 10mg
Phosphorus: 25mg
Sodium: 150mg

Lucky Charms:
Potassium: 25mg
Phosphorus: 40mg
Sodium: 210mg

Cinnamon Toast Crunch:
Potassium: 55mg
Phosphorus: 55mg
Sodium: 230mg

Cap'n Crunch:
Potassium: 20mg
Phosphorus: 50mg
Sodium: 180mg

Frosted Mini-Wheats:
Potassium: 190mg
Phosphorus: 120mg
Sodium: 0mg

Apple Jacks:
Potassium: 25mg
Phosphorus: 40mg
Sodium: 140mg

Quaker Oatmeal Squares:
Potassium: 115mg
Phosphorus: 100mg
Sodium: 170mg

Cinnamon Life:
Potassium: 115mg
Phosphorus: 70mg
Sodium: 170mg

Honey Bunches of Oats:
Potassium: 115mg
Phosphorus: 90mg
Sodium: 160mg

Corn Pops:
Potassium: 20mg
Phosphorus: 40mg
Sodium: 130mg

Reese's Puffs:
Potassium: 55mg
Phosphorus: 55mg
Sodium: 240mg

Mini-Wheats:
Potassium: 190mg
Phosphorus: 120mg

Sodium: 0mg

Rice Chex:
Potassium: 20mg
Phosphorus: 20mg
Sodium: 230mg

Fruity Pebbles:
Potassium: 10mg
Phosphorus: 25mg
Sodium: 150mg

Grape-Nuts:
Potassium: 280mg
Phosphorus: 250mg
Sodium: 290mg

Bran Flakes:
Potassium: 210mg
Phosphorus: 110mg
Sodium: 190mg

Honeycomb:
Potassium: 20mg
Phosphorus: 40mg
Sodium: 130mg

Kix:
Potassium: 20mg
Phosphorus: 40mg
Sodium: 190mg

Multi Grain Cheerios:
Potassium: 115mg
Phosphorus: 70mg
Sodium: 160mg

Shredded Wheat:
Potassium: 120mg
Phosphorus: 100mg
Sodium: 0mg

Frosted Shredded Wheat:
Potassium: 120mg
Phosphorus: 100mg
Sodium: 0mg

Bran Flakes:
Potassium: 210mg
Phosphorus: 110mg
Sodium: 190mg

Alpha-Bits:
Potassium: 20mg
Phosphorus: 40mg
Sodium: 200mg

Honey Graham Oh's:
Potassium: 35mg
Phosphorus: 50mg
Sodium: 170mg

Golden Grahams:
Potassium: 55mg
Phosphorus: 55mg

Sodium: 220mg

Fruity Cheerios:
Potassium: 115mg
Phosphorus: 70mg
Sodium: 160mg

Rice Krispies Treats Cereal:
Potassium: 20mg
Phosphorus: 30mg
Sodium: 130mg

Corn Bran:
Potassium: 80mg
Phosphorus: 60mg
Sodium: 210mg

Corn Puffs:
Potassium: 10mg
Phosphorus: 20mg
Sodium: 150mg

Cinnamon Graham Crunch:
Potassium: 35mg
Phosphorus: 50mg
Sodium: 170mg

Waffle Crisp:
Potassium: 20mg
Phosphorus: 35mg
Sodium: 150mg

Apple Cinnamon Cheerios:
Potassium: 115mg
Phosphorus: 70mg
Sodium: 160mg

Cookie Crisp:
Potassium: 35mg
Phosphorus: 45mg
Sodium: 200mg

Rice Krispies with Marshmallows:
Potassium: 20mg
Phosphorus: 30mg
Sodium: 200mg

Oreo O's:
Potassium: 45mg
Phosphorus: 45mg
Sodium: 180mg

Honey Smacks:
Potassium: 20mg
Phosphorus: 40mg
Sodium: 160mg

Krave:
Potassium: 55mg
Phosphorus: 55mg
Sodium: 240mg

Trix:
Potassium: 25mg
Phosphorus: 40mg

Sodium: 160mg

Oat Bran:
Potassium: 160mg
Phosphorus: 170mg
Sodium: 5mg

Corn Bran:
Potassium: 80mg
Phosphorus: 60mg
Sodium: 210mg

Maple Brown Sugar Crunch:
Potassium: 35mg
Phosphorus: 55mg
Sodium: 170mg

Granola:
Potassium: 140mg
Phosphorus: 80mg
Sodium: 5mg

Dairy and Dairy Alternatives

Whole Milk (1 cup):
Potassium: 366mg
Phosphorus: 247mg
Sodium: 98mg

Skim Milk (1 cup):
Potassium: 382mg
Phosphorus: 247mg
Sodium: 126mg

2% Milk (1 cup):
Potassium: 366mg
Phosphorus: 247mg
Sodium: 102mg

Soy Milk (1 cup):
Potassium: 300mg
Phosphorus: 80mg
Sodium: 100mg

Almond Milk (1 cup):
Potassium: 190mg
Phosphorus: 20mg
Sodium: 160mg

Rice Milk (1 cup):
Potassium: 10mg
Phosphorus: 30mg
Sodium: 90mg

Coconut Milk (1 cup):
Potassium: 497mg
Phosphorus: 48mg
Sodium: 15mg

Goat Milk (1 cup):
Potassium: 498mg
Phosphorus: 325mg
Sodium: 122mg

Sheep Milk (1 cup):
Potassium: 467mg
Phosphorus: 381mg

Sodium: 186mg

Cashew Milk (1 cup):
Potassium: 160mg
Phosphorus: 45mg
Sodium: 130mg

Hemp Milk (1 cup):
Potassium: 140mg
Phosphorus: 170mg
Sodium: 140mg

Oat Milk (1 cup):
Potassium: 120mg
Phosphorus: 90mg
Sodium: 100mg

Greek Yogurt (6 oz):
Potassium: 240mg
Phosphorus: 200mg
Sodium: 70mg

Plain Yogurt (6 oz):
Potassium: 250mg
Phosphorus: 200mg
Sodium: 80mg

Low-fat Yogurt (6 oz):
Potassium: 290mg
Phosphorus: 210mg
Sodium: 85mg

Non-fat Yogurt (6 oz):
Potassium: 270mg
Phosphorus: 200mg
Sodium: 85mg

Kefir (1 cup):
Potassium: 380mg
Phosphorus: 300mg
Sodium: 120mg

Cottage Cheese (1/2 cup):
Potassium: 80mg
Phosphorus: 92mg
Sodium: 370mg

Ricotta Cheese (1/2 cup):
Potassium: 126mg
Phosphorus: 189mg
Sodium: 210mg

Cheddar Cheese (1 oz):
Potassium: 27mg
Phosphorus: 121mg
Sodium: 174mg

Swiss Cheese (1 oz):
Potassium: 50mg
Phosphorus: 86mg
Sodium: 55mg

Feta Cheese (1 oz):
Potassium: 14mg
Phosphorus: 63mg

Sodium: 316mg

Parmesan Cheese (1 tbsp):
Potassium: 12mg
Phosphorus: 20mg
Sodium: 76mg

Mozzarella Cheese (1 oz):
Potassium: 18mg
Phosphorus: 82mg
Sodium: 138mg

Goat Cheese (1 oz):
Potassium: 20mg
Phosphorus: 42mg
Sodium: 100mg

Blue Cheese (1 oz):
Potassium: 26mg
Phosphorus: 52mg
Sodium: 325mg

Brie Cheese (1 oz):
Potassium: 36mg
Phosphorus: 45mg
Sodium: 178mg

American Cheese (1 oz):
Potassium: 23mg
Phosphorus: 153mg
Sodium: 406mg

Cream Cheese (1 oz):
Potassium: 14mg
Phosphorus: 32mg
Sodium: 123mg

Sour Cream (2 tbsp):
Potassium: 44mg
Phosphorus: 19mg
Sodium: 11mg

Whipped Cream (1 tbsp):
Potassium: 5mg
Phosphorus: 2mg
Sodium: 1mg

Evaporated Milk (1 cup):
Potassium: 730mg
Phosphorus: 550mg
Sodium: 420mg

Condensed Milk (1 cup):
Potassium: 911mg
Phosphorus: 600mg
Sodium: 282mg

Chocolate Milk (1 cup):
Potassium: 366mg
Phosphorus: 417mg
Sodium: 165mg

Buttermilk (1 cup):
Potassium: 370mg
Phosphorus: 250mg

Sodium: 260mg

Half and Half (1 tbsp):
Potassium: 22mg
Phosphorus: 20mg
Sodium: 6mg

Eggnog (1 cup):
Potassium: 275mg
Phosphorus: 210mg
Sodium: 180mg

Chocolate Almond Milk (1 cup):
Potassium: 210mg
Phosphorus: 180mg
Sodium: 160mg

Strawberry Milk (1 cup):
Potassium: 366mg
Phosphorus: 305mg
Sodium: 156mg

Vanilla Soy Milk (1 cup):
Potassium: 300mg
Phosphorus: 120mg
Sodium: 100mg

Hazelnut Milk (1 cup):
Potassium: 50mg
Phosphorus: 20mg
Sodium: 150mg

Goat Milk Yogurt (6 oz):
Potassium: 498mg
Phosphorus: 325mg
Sodium: 122mg

Sheep Milk Yogurt (6 oz):
Potassium: 467mg
Phosphorus: 381mg
Sodium: 186mg

Greek-style Goat Milk Yogurt (6 oz):
Potassium: 240mg
Phosphorus: 200mg
Sodium: 70mg

Greek-style Sheep Milk Yogurt (6 oz):
Potassium: 240mg
Phosphorus: 200mg
Sodium: 70mg

Soy Greek-style Yogurt (6 oz):
Potassium: 240mg
Phosphorus: 80mg
Sodium: 70mg

Almond Greek-style Yogurt (6 oz):
Potassium: 190mg
Phosphorus: 20mg
Sodium: 70mg

Coconut Greek-style Yogurt (6 oz):
Potassium: 250mg
Phosphorus: 20mg

Sodium: 30mg

Goat Cheese Spread (1 oz):
Potassium: 20mg
Phosphorus: 42mg
Sodium: 100mg

Sheep Cheese Spread (1 oz):
Potassium: 20mg
Phosphorus: 42mg
Sodium: 100mg

Dressings, Fats, and Oils

Olive Oil (1 tbsp):
Potassium: 0mg
Phosphorus: 0mg
Sodium: 0mg

Canola Oil (1 tbsp):
Potassium: 0mg
Phosphorus: 0mg
Sodium: 0mg

Vegetable Oil (1 tbsp):
Potassium: 0mg
Phosphorus: 0mg
Sodium: 0mg

Coconut Oil (1 tbsp):
Potassium: 0mg
Phosphorus: 0mg
Sodium: 0mg

Avocado Oil (1 tbsp):
Potassium: 0mg
Phosphorus: 0mg
Sodium: 0mg

Sesame Oil (1 tbsp):
Potassium: 0mg
Phosphorus: 0mg
Sodium: 0mg

Sunflower Oil (1 tbsp):
Potassium: 0mg
Phosphorus: 0mg
Sodium: 0mg

Flaxseed Oil (1 tbsp):
Potassium: 0mg
Phosphorus: 0mg
Sodium: 0mg

Walnut Oil (1 tbsp):
Potassium: 0mg
Phosphorus: 0mg
Sodium: 0mg

Grapeseed Oil (1 tbsp):
Potassium: 0mg
Phosphorus: 0mg
Sodium: 0mg

Butter (1 tbsp):
Potassium: 12mg
Phosphorus: 6mg

Sodium: 31mg

Margarine (1 tbsp):
Potassium: 8mg
Phosphorus: 3mg
Sodium: 101mg

Mayonnaise (1 tbsp):
Potassium: 1mg
Phosphorus: 2mg
Sodium: 78mg

Ranch Dressing (1 tbsp):
Potassium: 3mg
Phosphorus: 4mg
Sodium: 144mg

Caesar Dressing (1 tbsp):
Potassium: 2mg
Phosphorus: 4mg
Sodium: 130mg

Italian Dressing (1 tbsp):
Potassium: 7mg
Phosphorus: 3mg
Sodium: 149mg

Balsamic Vinaigrette (1 tbsp):
Potassium: 5mg
Phosphorus: 2mg
Sodium: 68mg

Thousand Island Dressing (1 tbsp):
Potassium: 10mg
Phosphorus: 3mg
Sodium: 70mg

Blue Cheese Dressing (1 tbsp):
Potassium: 5mg
Phosphorus: 4mg
Sodium: 154mg

French Dressing (1 tbsp):
Potassium: 11mg
Phosphorus: 3mg
Sodium: 115mg

Peanut Oil (1 tbsp):
Potassium: 0mg
Phosphorus: 0mg
Sodium: 0mg

Soybean Oil (1 tbsp):
Potassium: 0mg
Phosphorus: 0mg
Sodium: 0mg

Safflower Oil (1 tbsp):
Potassium: 0mg
Phosphorus: 0mg
Sodium: 0mg

Corn Oil (1 tbsp):
Potassium: 0mg
Phosphorus: 0mg

Sodium: 0mg

Hemp Oil (1 tbsp):
Potassium: 0mg
Phosphorus: 0mg
Sodium: 0mg

Duck Fat (1 tbsp):
Potassium: 0mg
Phosphorus: 0mg
Sodium: 0mg

Goose Fat (1 tbsp):
Potassium: 0mg
Phosphorus: 0mg
Sodium: 0mg

Bacon Fat (1 tbsp):
Potassium: 0mg
Phosphorus: 0mg
Sodium: 12mg

Ghee (1 tbsp):
Potassium: 1mg
Phosphorus: 1mg
Sodium: 2mg

Tahini (1 tbsp):
Potassium: 42mg
Phosphorus: 27mg
Sodium: 42mg

Walnut Butter (1 tbsp):
Potassium: 40mg
Phosphorus: 25mg
Sodium: 1mg

Almond Butter (1 tbsp):
Potassium: 90mg
Phosphorus: 50mg
Sodium: 0mg

Cashew Butter (1 tbsp):
Potassium: 60mg
Phosphorus: 80mg
Sodium: 0mg

Sunflower Seed Butter (1 tbsp):
Potassium: 65mg
Phosphorus: 70mg
Sodium: 0mg

Coconut Butter (1 tbsp):
Potassium: 50mg
Phosphorus: 10mg
Sodium: 0mg

Soybean Butter (1 tbsp):
Potassium: 46mg
Phosphorus: 79mg
Sodium: 81mg

Sesame Seed Butter (Tahini) (1 tbsp):
Potassium: 44mg
Phosphorus: 27mg

Sodium: 42mg

Olive Tapenade (1 tbsp):
Potassium: 14mg
Phosphorus: 5mg
Sodium: 215mg

Pesto Sauce (1 tbsp):
Potassium: 25mg
Phosphorus: 12mg
Sodium: 100mg

Hummus (1 tbsp):
Potassium: 11mg
Phosphorus: 4mg
Sodium: 35mg

Guacamole (1 tbsp):
Potassium: 46mg
Phosphorus: 5mg
Sodium: 42mg

Creamy Salad Dressing (1 tbsp):
Potassium: 3mg
Phosphorus: 4mg
Sodium: 45mg

Poppy Seed Dressing (1 tbsp):
Potassium: 6mg
Phosphorus: 4mg
Sodium: 35mg

Sesame Seed Dressing (1 tbsp):

Potassium: 7mg
Phosphorus: 5mg
Sodium: 85mg

Lemon Vinaigrette (1 tbsp):
Potassium: 16mg
Phosphorus: 2mg
Sodium: 62mg

Lime Vinaigrette (1 tbsp):
Potassium: 6mg
Phosphorus: 2mg
Sodium: 59mg

Raspberry Vinaigrette (1 tbsp):
Potassium: 10mg
Phosphorus: 2mg
Sodium: 85mg

Apple Cider Vinegar Dressing (1 tbsp):
Potassium: 11mg
Phosphorus: 0mg
Sodium: 5mg

White Wine Vinaigrette (1 tbsp):
Potassium: 3mg
Phosphorus: 2mg
Sodium: 41mg

Red Wine Vinaigrette (1 tbsp):
Potassium: 6mg
Phosphorus: 2mg
Sodium: 55mg

McDonald's Big Mac:
Potassium: 360mg
Phosphorus: 310mg
Sodium: 970mg

Burger King Whopper:
Potassium: 290mg
Phosphorus: 280mg
Sodium: 980mg

Wendy's Baconator:
Potassium: 450mg
Phosphorus: 420mg
Sodium: 1330mg

Taco Bell Crunchy Taco:
Potassium: 220mg
Phosphorus: 170mg
Sodium: 390mg

Subway 6-inch Turkey Breast Sandwich:
Potassium: 310mg
Phosphorus: 270mg
Sodium: 830mg

KFC Original Recipe Chicken Breast:
Potassium: 380mg
Phosphorus: 300mg
Sodium: 1130mg

Pizza Hut Pepperoni Pizza (1 slice):
Potassium: 130mg
Phosphorus: 75mg
Sodium: 340mg

Domino's Cheese Pizza (1 slice):
Potassium: 80mg
Phosphorus: 65mg
Sodium: 190mg

Chipotle Chicken Burrito Bowl:
Potassium: 660mg
Phosphorus: 410mg
Sodium: 1160mg

Chick-fil-A Chicken Sandwich:
Potassium: 320mg
Phosphorus: 270mg
Sodium: 1350mg

Dunkin' Donuts Glazed Donut:
Potassium: 45mg
Phosphorus: 70mg
Sodium: 130mg

Starbucks Caffe Latte (Tall):
Potassium: 340mg
Phosphorus: 220mg
Sodium: 150mg

Panda Express Orange Chicken:
Potassium: 240mg
Phosphorus: 130mg

Sodium: 880mg

Dairy Queen Cheeseburger:
Potassium: 330mg
Phosphorus: 220mg
Sodium: 850mg

Jack in the Box Jumbo Jack:
Potassium: 340mg
Phosphorus: 260mg
Sodium: 770mg

Carl's Jr. Famous Star Burger:
Potassium: 310mg
Phosphorus: 280mg
Sodium: 860mg

Popeyes Chicken Sandwich:
Potassium: 330mg
Phosphorus: 200mg
Sodium: 1390mg

In-N-Out Double-Double Burger:
Potassium: 360mg
Phosphorus: 300mg
Sodium: 1440mg

Sonic Drive-In Cheeseburger:
Potassium: 270mg
Phosphorus: 220mg
Sodium: 780mg

Arby's Classic Roast Beef Sandwich:
Potassium: 420mg
Phosphorus: 330mg
Sodium: 970mg

Five Guys Hamburger:
Potassium: 370mg
Phosphorus: 310mg
Sodium: 520mg

Pizza Hut Breadsticks (2 pieces):
Potassium: 35mg
Phosphorus: 20mg
Sodium: 240mg

Domino's Chicken Wings (4 pieces):
Potassium: 80mg
Phosphorus: 90mg
Sodium: 360mg

Subway Meatball Marinara Sub (6-inch):
Potassium: 260mg
Phosphorus: 240mg
Sodium: 940mg

Taco Bell Bean Burrito:
Potassium: 370mg
Phosphorus: 250mg
Sodium: 980mg

McDonald's Chicken McNuggets (6 pieces):
Potassium: 230mg
Phosphorus: 160mg

Sodium: 510mg

Burger King Chicken Fries (9 pieces):
Potassium: 180mg
Phosphorus: 210mg
Sodium: 1030mg

Wendy's Spicy Chicken Sandwich:
Potassium: 310mg
Phosphorus: 220mg
Sodium: 1020mg

KFC Popcorn Chicken (Large):
Potassium: 580mg
Phosphorus: 470mg
Sodium: 1750mg

Chick-fil-A Spicy Deluxe Sandwich:
Potassium: 320mg
Phosphorus: 270mg
Sodium: 1580mg

Dunkin' Donuts Bacon, Egg & Cheese Croissant:
Potassium: 140mg
Phosphorus: 280mg
Sodium: 890mg

Starbucks Mocha Frappuccino (Tall):
Potassium: 210mg
Phosphorus: 180mg
Sodium: 180mg

Panda Express Beef with Broccoli:
Potassium: 400mg
Phosphorus: 200mg
Sodium: 1070mg

Dairy Queen Chicken Strip Basket:
Potassium: 340mg
Phosphorus: 210mg
Sodium: 1090mg

Jack in the Box Ultimate Cheeseburger:
Potassium: 290mg
Phosphorus: 270mg
Sodium: 1180mg

Carl's Jr. Western Bacon Cheeseburger:
Potassium: 280mg
Phosphorus: 270mg
Sodium: 1140mg

Popeyes Spicy Chicken Tenders (5 pieces):
Potassium: 220mg
Phosphorus: 150mg
Sodium: 1230mg

In-N-Out Animal Style Fries:
Potassium: 490mg
Phosphorus: 130mg
Sodium: 1510mg

Sonic Drive-In Chili Cheese Coney:
Potassium: 330mg
Phosphorus: 200mg

Sodium: 1150mg

Arby's Loaded Italian Sub:
Potassium: 340mg
Phosphorus: 220mg
Sodium: 1710mg

Five Guys Bacon Cheeseburger:
Potassium: 380mg
Phosphorus: 280mg
Sodium: 1140mg

Pizza Hut Stuffed Crust Pizza (1 slice):
Potassium: 80mg
Phosphorus: 60mg
Sodium: 310mg

Domino's Chocolate Lava Crunch Cake:
Potassium: 50mg
Phosphorus: 60mg
Sodium: 140mg

Subway Spicy Italian Sub (6-inch):
Potassium: 250mg
Phosphorus: 220mg
Sodium: 990mg

Taco Bell Cheesy Gordita Crunch:
Potassium: 220mg
Phosphorus: 170mg
Sodium: 490mg

McDonald's Filet-O-Fish Sandwich:
Potassium: 300mg
Phosphorus: 250mg
Sodium: 580mg

Burger King Chicken Nuggets (10 pieces):
Potassium: 360mg
Phosphorus: 300mg
Sodium: 1260mg

Wendy's Jr. Bacon Cheeseburger:
Potassium: 270mg
Phosphorus: 240mg
Sodium: 730mg

KFC Crispy Chicken Sandwich:
Potassium: 310mg
Phosphorus: 280mg
Sodium: 820mg

Chick-fil-A Grilled Chicken Sandwich:
Potassium: 320mg
Phosphorus: 270mg
Sodium: 990mg

Fruits and Fruit Products

Apple (1 medium):
Potassium: 195mg
Phosphorus: 20mg
Sodium: 2mg

Banana (1 medium):
Potassium: 422mg
Phosphorus: 26mg
Sodium: 1mg

Orange (1 medium):
Potassium: 237mg
Phosphorus: 14mg
Sodium: 0mg

Strawberry (1 cup, sliced):
Potassium: 233mg
Phosphorus: 24mg
Sodium: 2mg

Blueberry (1 cup):
Potassium: 114mg
Phosphorus: 18mg
Sodium: 1mg

Watermelon (1 cup, diced):
Potassium: 170mg
Phosphorus: 15mg
Sodium: 3mg

Grapes (1 cup):
Potassium: 288mg
Phosphorus: 30mg
Sodium: 3mg

Pineapple (1 cup, diced):
Potassium: 180mg
Phosphorus: 13mg
Sodium: 2mg

Mango (1 cup, sliced):
Potassium: 277mg
Phosphorus: 20mg
Sodium: 3mg

Kiwi (1 medium):
Potassium: 252mg
Phosphorus: 26mg
Sodium: 3mg

Peach (1 medium):
Potassium: 285mg
Phosphorus: 20mg
Sodium: 0mg

Pear (1 medium):
Potassium: 190mg
Phosphorus: 15mg
Sodium: 1mg

Plum (1 medium):
Potassium: 113mg
Phosphorus: 11mg

Sodium: 0mg

Cherry (1 cup):
Potassium: 306mg
Phosphorus: 31mg
Sodium: 3mg

Raspberry (1 cup):
Potassium: 186mg
Phosphorus: 29mg
Sodium: 1mg

Blackberry (1 cup):
Potassium: 233mg
Phosphorus: 22mg
Sodium: 1mg

Cranberry (1 cup, whole):
Potassium: 195mg
Phosphorus: 13mg
Sodium: 2mg

Lemon (1 medium):
Potassium: 80mg
Phosphorus: 10mg
Sodium: 1mg

Lime (1 medium):
Potassium: 68mg
Phosphorus: 12mg
Sodium: 0mg

Grapefruit (1 medium):
Potassium: 332mg
Phosphorus: 20mg
Sodium: 0mg

Apricot (1 medium):
Potassium: 259mg
Phosphorus: 20mg
Sodium: 1mg

Papaya (1 cup, diced):
Potassium: 360mg
Phosphorus: 20mg
Sodium: 11mg

Cantaloupe (1 cup, diced):
Potassium: 473mg
Phosphorus: 29mg
Sodium: 28mg

Honeydew Melon (1 cup, diced):
Potassium: 388mg
Phosphorus: 30mg
Sodium: 30mg

Fig (1 medium):
Potassium: 232mg
Phosphorus: 20mg
Sodium: 1mg

Date (1 medium):
Potassium: 167mg
Phosphorus: 62mg

Sodium: 0mg

Passion Fruit (1 medium):
Potassium: 229mg
Phosphorus: 68mg
Sodium: 28mg

Guava (1 medium):
Potassium: 688mg
Phosphorus: 66mg
Sodium: 3mg

Lychee (1 cup):
Potassium: 325mg
Phosphorus: 31mg
Sodium: 1mg

Tangerine (1 medium):
Potassium: 166mg
Phosphorus: 14mg
Sodium: 2mg

Persimmon (1 medium):
Potassium: 270mg
Phosphorus: 34mg
Sodium: 0mg

Nectarine (1 medium):
Potassium: 285mg
Phosphorus: 26mg
Sodium: 0mg

Pomegranate (1 medium):
Potassium: 666mg
Phosphorus: 28mg
Sodium: 5mg

Kiwifruit (1 medium):
Potassium: 237mg
Phosphorus: 30mg
Sodium: 3mg

Starfruit (1 medium):
Potassium: 176mg
Phosphorus: 17mg
Sodium: 3mg

Mulberry (1 cup):
Potassium: 272mg
Phosphorus: 39mg
Sodium: 10mg

Elderberry (1 cup):
Potassium: 406mg
Phosphorus: 58mg
Sodium: 4mg

Ackee (1 cup):
Potassium: 920mg
Phosphorus: 250mg
Sodium: 4mg

Ugli Fruit (1 medium):
Potassium: 324mg
Phosphorus: 51mg

Sodium: 4mg

Longan (1 cup):
Potassium: 285mg
Phosphorus: 33mg
Sodium: 1mg

Plantain (1 medium):
Potassium: 893mg
Phosphorus: 66mg
Sodium: 2mg

Breadfruit (1 cup, sliced):
Potassium: 490mg
Phosphorus: 44mg
Sodium: 2mg

Cherimoya (1 medium):
Potassium: 839mg
Phosphorus: 287mg
Sodium: 7mg

Carambola (1 medium):
Potassium: 133mg
Phosphorus: 29mg
Sodium: 2mg

Pomelo (1 cup, sections):
Potassium: 397mg
Phosphorus: 34mg
Sodium: 3mg

Jabuticaba (1 cup):

Potassium: 325mg
Phosphorus: 23mg
Sodium: 3mg

Guanabana (1 cup, pureed):
Potassium: 645mg
Phosphorus: 62mg
Sodium: 0mg

Feijoa (1 medium):
Potassium: 241mg
Phosphorus: 22mg
Sodium: 1mg

Tamarillo (1 medium):
Potassium: 288mg
Phosphorus: 39mg
Sodium: 3mg

Durian (1 cup):
Potassium: 1056mg
Phosphorus: 105mg
Sodium: 3mg

Salmon (3 oz, cooked):
Potassium: 366mg
Phosphorus: 281mg
Sodium: 50mg

Tuna (3 oz, canned in water):
Potassium: 201mg
Phosphorus: 200mg
Sodium: 255mg

Cod (3 oz, cooked):
Potassium: 439mg
Phosphorus: 234mg
Sodium: 78mg

Trout (3 oz, cooked):
Potassium: 354mg
Phosphorus: 208mg
Sodium: 53mg

Sardines (3 oz, canned in water):
Potassium: 325mg
Phosphorus: 300mg
Sodium: 200mg

Halibut (3 oz, cooked):
Potassium: 490mg
Phosphorus: 271mg
Sodium: 70mg

Haddock (3 oz, cooked):
Potassium: 474mg

Phosphorus: 260mg
Sodium: 99mg

Mackerel (3 oz, cooked):
Potassium: 360mg
Phosphorus: 263mg
Sodium: 90mg

Tilapia (3 oz, cooked):
Potassium: 335mg
Phosphorus: 204mg
Sodium: 51mg

Shrimp (3 oz, cooked):
Potassium: 190mg
Phosphorus: 222mg
Sodium: 247mg

Crab (3 oz, cooked):
Potassium: 286mg
Phosphorus: 186mg
Sodium: 273mg

Lobster (3 oz, cooked):
Potassium: 286mg
Phosphorus: 187mg
Sodium: 719mg

Scallops (3 oz, cooked):
Potassium: 314mg
Phosphorus: 290mg
Sodium: 480mg

Clams (3 oz, cooked):
Potassium: 534mg
Phosphorus: 228mg
Sodium: 78mg

Oysters (3 oz, cooked):
Potassium: 270mg
Phosphorus: 205mg
Sodium: 207mg

Anchovies (3 oz, canned in oil):
Potassium: 192mg
Phosphorus: 222mg
Sodium: 351mg

Catfish (3 oz, cooked):
Potassium: 367mg
Phosphorus: 194mg
Sodium: 70mg

Swordfish (3 oz, cooked):
Potassium: 314mg
Phosphorus: 248mg
Sodium: 92mg

Mahi Mahi (3 oz, cooked):
Potassium: 377mg
Phosphorus: 266mg
Sodium: 87mg

Sole (3 oz, cooked):
Potassium: 458mg
Phosphorus: 260mg

Sodium: 78mg

Herring (3 oz, cooked):
Potassium: 435mg
Phosphorus: 390mg
Sodium: 63mg

Pollock (3 oz, cooked):
Potassium: 436mg
Phosphorus: 259mg
Sodium: 83mg

Perch (3 oz, cooked):
Potassium: 370mg
Phosphorus: 249mg
Sodium: 56mg

Red Snapper (3 oz, cooked):
Potassium: 345mg
Phosphorus: 250mg
Sodium: 76mg

Grouper (3 oz, cooked):
Potassium: 520mg
Phosphorus: 223mg
Sodium: 99mg

Rockfish (3 oz, cooked):
Potassium: 360mg
Phosphorus: 262mg
Sodium: 89mg

Canned Tuna (3 oz, canned in oil):
Potassium: 196mg
Phosphorus: 200mg
Sodium: 339mg

Squid (3 oz, cooked):
Potassium: 384mg
Phosphorus: 226mg
Sodium: 145mg

Eel (3 oz, cooked):
Potassium: 221mg
Phosphorus: 241mg
Sodium: 116mg

Tilapia (3 oz, cooked):
Potassium: 186mg
Phosphorus: 204mg
Sodium: 51mg

Tuna Steak (3 oz, cooked):
Potassium: 339mg
Phosphorus: 239mg
Sodium: 53mg

Rainbow Trout (3 oz, cooked):
Potassium: 334mg
Phosphorus: 207mg
Sodium: 53mg

Arctic Char (3 oz, cooked):
Potassium: 330mg
Phosphorus: 192mg

Sodium: 66mg

Smelt (3 oz, cooked):
Potassium: 309mg
Phosphorus: 244mg
Sodium: 74mg

Tilapia (3 oz, cooked):
Potassium: 335mg
Phosphorus: 204mg
Sodium: 51mg

Canned Salmon (3 oz, canned in water):
Potassium: 265mg
Phosphorus: 296mg
Sodium: 44mg

Mussels (3 oz, cooked):
Potassium: 384mg
Phosphorus: 302mg
Sodium: 336mg

Herring Roe (3 oz, cooked):
Potassium: 447mg
Phosphorus: 615mg
Sodium: 96mg

Monkfish (3 oz, cooked):
Potassium: 404mg
Phosphorus: 207mg
Sodium: 94mg

Cuttlefish (3 oz, cooked):
Potassium: 339mg
Phosphorus: 194mg
Sodium: 131mg

Marlin (3 oz, cooked):
Potassium: 315mg
Phosphorus: 190mg
Sodium: 64mg

Alaska Pollock (3 oz, cooked):
Potassium: 420mg
Phosphorus: 197mg
Sodium: 97mg

Tilapia (3 oz, cooked):
Potassium: 335mg
Phosphorus: 204mg
Sodium: 51mg

Whitefish (3 oz, cooked):
Potassium: 393mg
Phosphorus: 191mg
Sodium: 79mg

Abalone (3 oz, cooked):
Potassium: 959mg
Phosphorus: 557mg
Sodium: 236mg

Sturgeon (3 oz, cooked):
Potassium: 405mg
Phosphorus: 228mg

Sodium: 72mg

Hoki (3 oz, cooked):
Potassium: 420mg
Phosphorus: 207mg
Sodium: 97mg

Orange Roughy (3 oz, cooked):
Potassium: 436mg
Phosphorus: 203mg
Sodium: 55mg

Tuna Salad (1 cup):
Potassium: 245mg
Phosphorus: 265mg
Sodium: 421mg

Smoked Salmon (3 oz):
Potassium: 297mg
Phosphorus: 283mg
Sodium: 876mg

Grains and Pasta

White Rice (1/2 cup, cooked):
Potassium: 35mg
Phosphorus: 32mg
Sodium: 1mg

Brown Rice (1/2 cup, cooked):
Potassium: 86mg
Phosphorus: 76mg
Sodium: 2mg

Quinoa (1/2 cup, cooked):
Potassium: 118mg
Phosphorus: 118mg
Sodium: 7mg

Bulgur (1/2 cup, cooked):
Potassium: 59mg
Phosphorus: 65mg
Sodium: 1mg

Millet (1/2 cup, cooked):
Potassium: 66mg
Phosphorus: 82mg
Sodium: 2mg

Barley (1/2 cup, cooked):
Potassium: 97mg
Phosphorus: 63mg
Sodium: 1mg

Buckwheat (1/2 cup, cooked):
Potassium: 91mg

Phosphorus: 87mg
Sodium: 1mg

Farro (1/2 cup, cooked):
Potassium: 83mg
Phosphorus: 66mg
Sodium: 2mg

Couscous (1/2 cup, cooked):
Potassium: 58mg
Phosphorus: 55mg
Sodium: 1mg

Oats (1/2 cup, cooked):
Potassium: 78mg
Phosphorus: 95mg
Sodium: 1mg

Whole Wheat Pasta (1/2 cup, cooked):
Potassium: 50mg
Phosphorus: 67mg
Sodium: 1mg

Spaghetti (1/2 cup, cooked):
Potassium: 43mg
Phosphorus: 34mg
Sodium: 1mg

Macaroni (1/2 cup, cooked):
Potassium: 39mg
Phosphorus: 33mg
Sodium: 1mg

Egg Noodles (1/2 cup, cooked):
Potassium: 38mg
Phosphorus: 30mg
Sodium: 1mg

Angel Hair Pasta (1/2 cup, cooked):
Potassium: 38mg
Phosphorus: 33mg
Sodium: 1mg

Linguine (1/2 cup, cooked):
Potassium: 43mg
Phosphorus: 36mg
Sodium: 1mg

Vermicelli (1/2 cup, cooked):
Potassium: 43mg
Phosphorus: 36mg
Sodium: 1mg

Fettuccine (1/2 cup, cooked):
Potassium: 43mg
Phosphorus: 36mg
Sodium: 1mg

Orzo (1/2 cup, cooked):
Potassium: 33mg
Phosphorus: 28mg
Sodium: 1mg

Rotini (1/2 cup, cooked):
Potassium: 39mg
Phosphorus: 33mg

Sodium: 1mg

Penne (1/2 cup, cooked):
Potassium: 39mg
Phosphorus: 33mg
Sodium: 1mg

Rigatoni (1/2 cup, cooked):
Potassium: 39mg
Phosphorus: 33mg
Sodium: 1mg

Lasagna (1/2 cup, cooked):
Potassium: 39mg
Phosphorus: 33mg
Sodium: 1mg

Pearl Barley (1/2 cup, cooked):
Potassium: 97mg
Phosphorus: 63mg
Sodium: 1mg

Spelt (1/2 cup, cooked):
Potassium: 66mg
Phosphorus: 82mg
Sodium: 2mg

Wheat Berries (1/2 cup, cooked):
Potassium: 123mg
Phosphorus: 148mg
Sodium: 2mg

Rye (1/2 cup, cooked):
Potassium: 93mg
Phosphorus: 74mg
Sodium: 1mg

Teff (1/2 cup, cooked):
Potassium: 70mg
Phosphorus: 130mg
Sodium: 3mg

Sorghum (1/2 cup, cooked):
Potassium: 130mg
Phosphorus: 140mg
Sodium: 2mg

Rice Noodles (1/2 cup, cooked):
Potassium: 34mg
Phosphorus: 20mg
Sodium: 1mg

Polenta (1/2 cup, cooked):
Potassium: 40mg
Phosphorus: 60mg
Sodium: 1mg

Grits (1/2 cup, cooked):
Potassium: 44mg
Phosphorus: 24mg
Sodium: 125mg

Amaranth (1/2 cup, cooked):
Potassium: 116mg
Phosphorus: 150mg

Sodium: 1mg

Cornmeal (1/2 cup, cooked):
Potassium: 140mg
Phosphorus: 70mg
Sodium: 1mg

Triticale (1/2 cup, cooked):
Potassium: 85mg
Phosphorus: 77mg
Sodium: 1mg

Kamut (1/2 cup, cooked):
Potassium: 111mg
Phosphorus: 135mg
Sodium: 1mg

Fonio (1/2 cup, cooked):
Potassium: 79mg
Phosphorus: 98mg
Sodium: 1mg

Freekeh (1/2 cup, cooked):
Potassium: 99mg
Phosphorus: 110mg
Sodium: 7mg

Einkorn (1/2 cup, cooked):
Potassium: 114mg
Phosphorus: 180mg
Sodium: 2mg

Emmer (1/2 cup, cooked):
Potassium: 103mg
Phosphorus: 133mg
Sodium: 2mg

Bulgur (1/2 cup, cooked):
Potassium: 59mg
Phosphorus: 65mg
Sodium: 1mg

Kamut (1/2 cup, cooked):
Potassium: 111mg
Phosphorus: 135mg
Sodium: 1mg

Teff (1/2 cup, cooked):
Potassium: 70mg
Phosphorus: 130mg
Sodium: 3mg

Farro (1/2 cup, cooked):
Potassium: 83mg
Phosphorus: 66mg
Sodium: 2mg

Sorghum (1/2 cup, cooked):
Potassium: 130mg
Phosphorus: 140mg
Sodium: 2mg

Fonio (1/2 cup, cooked):
Potassium: 79mg
Phosphorus: 98mg

Sodium: 1mg

Freekeh (1/2 cup, cooked):
Potassium: 99mg
Phosphorus: 110mg
Sodium: 7mg

Einkorn (1/2 cup, cooked):
Potassium: 114mg
Phosphorus: 180mg
Sodium: 2mg

Emmer (1/2 cup, cooked):
Potassium: 103mg
Phosphorus: 133mg
Sodium: 2mg

Rye (1/2 cup, cooked):
Potassium: 93mg
Phosphorus: 74mg
Sodium: 1mg

Meat

Chicken Breast (3 oz, cooked):
Potassium: 256mg
Phosphorus: 256mg
Sodium: 74mg

Turkey Breast (3 oz, cooked):
Potassium: 218mg
Phosphorus: 229mg
Sodium: 74mg

Beef Sirloin (3 oz, cooked):
Potassium: 292mg
Phosphorus: 181mg
Sodium: 62mg

Pork Tenderloin (3 oz, cooked):
Potassium: 364mg
Phosphorus: 235mg
Sodium: 58mg

Lamb Leg (3 oz, cooked):
Potassium: 254mg
Phosphorus: 178mg
Sodium: 58mg

Veal Chop (3 oz, cooked):
Potassium: 315mg
Phosphorus: 222mg
Sodium: 67mg

Bison Steak (3 oz, cooked):
Potassium: 333mg

Phosphorus: 196mg
Sodium: 71mg

Deer Venison (3 oz, cooked):
Potassium: 253mg
Phosphorus: 219mg
Sodium: 74mg

Chicken Thigh (3 oz, cooked):
Potassium: 263mg
Phosphorus: 249mg
Sodium: 77mg

Turkey Thigh (3 oz, cooked):
Potassium: 243mg
Phosphorus: 243mg
Sodium: 74mg

Beef Ribeye (3 oz, cooked):
Potassium: 320mg
Phosphorus: 180mg
Sodium: 67mg

Pork Loin (3 oz, cooked):
Potassium: 323mg
Phosphorus: 235mg
Sodium: 59mg

Lamb Chop (3 oz, cooked):
Potassium: 271mg
Phosphorus: 185mg
Sodium: 62mg

Veal Cutlet (3 oz, cooked):
Potassium: 278mg
Phosphorus: 220mg
Sodium: 70mg

Bison Burger (3 oz, cooked):
Potassium: 307mg
Phosphorus: 180mg
Sodium: 73mg

Deer Steak (3 oz, cooked):
Potassium: 249mg
Phosphorus: 219mg
Sodium: 75mg

Ground Chicken (3 oz, cooked):
Potassium: 220mg
Phosphorus: 230mg
Sodium: 70mg

Ground Turkey (3 oz, cooked):
Potassium: 224mg
Phosphorus: 223mg
Sodium: 70mg

Ground Beef (3 oz, cooked):
Potassium: 267mg
Phosphorus: 203mg
Sodium: 75mg

Ground Pork (3 oz, cooked):
Potassium: 284mg
Phosphorus: 219mg

Sodium: 72mg

Ground Lamb (3 oz, cooked):
Potassium: 271mg
Phosphorus: 198mg
Sodium: 72mg

Ground Bison (3 oz, cooked):
Potassium: 296mg
Phosphorus: 197mg
Sodium: 75mg

Ground Venison (3 oz, cooked):
Potassium: 242mg
Phosphorus: 219mg
Sodium: 75mg

Chicken Wing (1 wing, cooked):
Potassium: 69mg
Phosphorus: 92mg
Sodium: 22mg

Turkey Wing (1 wing, cooked):
Potassium: 61mg
Phosphorus: 93mg
Sodium: 26mg

Beef Liver (3 oz, cooked):
Potassium: 324mg
Phosphorus: 354mg
Sodium: 71mg

Pork Liver (3 oz, cooked):
Potassium: 330mg
Phosphorus: 364mg
Sodium: 71mg

Lamb Liver (3 oz, cooked):
Potassium: 309mg
Phosphorus: 336mg
Sodium: 70mg

Veal Liver (3 oz, cooked):
Potassium: 329mg
Phosphorus: 336mg
Sodium: 72mg

Chicken Drumstick (1 drumstick, cooked):
Potassium: 130mg
Phosphorus: 112mg
Sodium: 50mg

Turkey Drumstick (1 drumstick, cooked):
Potassium: 131mg
Phosphorus: 121mg
Sodium: 55mg

Beef Heart (3 oz, cooked):
Potassium: 275mg
Phosphorus: 281mg
Sodium: 63mg

Pork Heart (3 oz, cooked):
Potassium: 291mg
Phosphorus: 292mg

Sodium: 62mg

Lamb Heart (3 oz, cooked):
Potassium: 269mg
Phosphorus: 272mg
Sodium: 61mg

Veal Heart (3 oz, cooked):
Potassium: 287mg
Phosphorus: 292mg
Sodium: 63mg

Chicken Liver (3 oz, cooked):
Potassium: 249mg
Phosphorus: 373mg
Sodium: 89mg

Turkey Liver (3 oz, cooked):
Potassium: 271mg
Phosphorus: 364mg
Sodium: 88mg

Beef Tongue (3 oz, cooked):
Potassium: 256mg
Phosphorus: 268mg
Sodium: 70mg

Pork Tongue (3 oz, cooked):
Potassium: 276mg
Phosphorus: 292mg
Sodium: 71mg

Lamb Tongue (3 oz, cooked):
Potassium: 253mg
Phosphorus: 268mg
Sodium: 70mg

Veal Tongue (3 oz, cooked):
Potassium: 273mg
Phosphorus: 292mg
Sodium: 72mg

Chicken Gizzard (3 oz, cooked):
Potassium: 204mg
Phosphorus: 324mg
Sodium: 142mg

Turkey Gizzard (3 oz, cooked):
Potassium: 211mg
Phosphorus: 292mg
Sodium: 142mg

Beef Kidney (3 oz, cooked):
Potassium: 290mg
Phosphorus: 370mg
Sodium: 79mg

Pork Kidney (3 oz, cooked):
Potassium: 318mg
Phosphorus: 405mg
Sodium: 83mg

Lamb Kidney (3 oz, cooked):
Potassium: 287mg
Phosphorus: 365mg

Sodium: 79mg

Veal Kidney (3 oz, cooked):
Potassium: 306mg
Phosphorus: 400mg
Sodium: 82mg

Chicken Feet (1 foot, cooked):
Potassium: 63mg
Phosphorus: 81mg
Sodium: 38mg

Turkey Feet (1 foot, cooked):
Potassium: 64mg
Phosphorus: 85mg
Sodium: 42mg

Chicken Skin (3 oz, cooked):
Potassium: 99mg
Phosphorus: 99mg
Sodium: 76mg

Nuts and Seeds

Almonds (1 oz, dry roasted):
Potassium: 206mg
Phosphorus: 137mg
Sodium: 0mg

Walnuts (1 oz, English):
Potassium: 125mg
Phosphorus: 98mg
Sodium: 1mg

Pistachios (1 oz, dry roasted):
Potassium: 291mg
Phosphorus: 139mg
Sodium: 0mg

Cashews (1 oz, dry roasted):
Potassium: 187mg
Phosphorus: 168mg
Sodium: 3mg

Pecans (1 oz, dry roasted):
Potassium: 116mg
Phosphorus: 74mg
Sodium: 0mg

Hazelnuts (1 oz, dry roasted):
Potassium: 193mg
Phosphorus: 139mg
Sodium: 0mg

Brazil Nuts (1 oz):
Potassium: 187mg

Phosphorus: 197mg
Sodium: 1mg

Macadamia Nuts (1 oz):
Potassium: 103mg
Phosphorus: 54mg
Sodium: 1mg

Pine Nuts (1 oz):
Potassium: 149mg
Phosphorus: 162mg
Sodium: 1mg

Chestnuts (1 oz, roasted):
Potassium: 184mg
Phosphorus: 90mg
Sodium: 1mg

Sunflower Seeds (1 oz, dry roasted):
Potassium: 161mg
Phosphorus: 207mg
Sodium: 2mg

Pumpkin Seeds (1 oz, roasted):
Potassium: 163mg
Phosphorus: 213mg
Sodium: 5mg

Sesame Seeds (1 oz):
Potassium: 116mg
Phosphorus: 160mg
Sodium: 3mg

Flaxseeds (1 oz):
Potassium: 186mg
Phosphorus: 186mg
Sodium: 6mg

Chia Seeds (1 oz):
Potassium: 115mg
Phosphorus: 174mg
Sodium: 5mg

Hemp Seeds (1 oz):
Potassium: 240mg
Phosphorus: 495mg
Sodium: 3mg

Poppy Seeds (1 oz):
Potassium: 114mg
Phosphorus: 136mg
Sodium: 4mg

Watermelon Seeds (1 oz, dried):
Potassium: 186mg
Phosphorus: 424mg
Sodium: 7mg

Soy Nuts (1 oz, roasted):
Potassium: 379mg
Phosphorus: 301mg
Sodium: 3mg

Peanuts (1 oz, dry roasted):
Potassium: 180mg
Phosphorus: 107mg

Sodium: 2mg

Cashew Butter (1 tbsp):
Potassium: 67mg
Phosphorus: 50mg
Sodium: 0mg

Almond Butter (1 tbsp):
Potassium: 98mg
Phosphorus: 43mg
Sodium: 0mg

Sunflower Butter (1 tbsp):
Potassium: 39mg
Phosphorus: 42mg
Sodium: 1mg

Tahini (1 tbsp):
Potassium: 79mg
Phosphorus: 37mg
Sodium: 1mg

Pumpkin Seed Butter (1 tbsp):
Potassium: 41mg
Phosphorus: 44mg
Sodium: 1mg

Flaxseed Butter (1 tbsp):
Potassium: 60mg
Phosphorus: 55mg
Sodium: 1mg

Chia Seed Butter (1 tbsp):
Potassium: 35mg
Phosphorus: 30mg
Sodium: 1mg

Coconut (1 oz, shredded):
Potassium: 101mg
Phosphorus: 49mg
Sodium: 7mg

Coconut Milk (1 cup):
Potassium: 497mg
Phosphorus: 178mg
Sodium: 13mg

Coconut Water (1 cup):
Potassium: 600mg
Phosphorus: 60mg
Sodium: 252mg

Coconut Cream (1 oz):
Potassium: 40mg
Phosphorus: 10mg
Sodium: 1mg

Coconut Oil (1 tbsp):
Potassium: 0mg
Phosphorus: 0mg
Sodium: 0mg

Coconut Flour (1 oz):
Potassium: 105mg
Phosphorus: 105mg

Sodium: 25mg

Coconut Sugar (1 tsp):
Potassium: 10mg
Phosphorus: 1mg
Sodium: 0mg

Coconut Aminos (1 tbsp):
Potassium: 90mg
Phosphorus: 10mg
Sodium: 160mg

Pine Nut Butter (1 tbsp):
Potassium: 34mg
Phosphorus: 36mg
Sodium: 1mg

Hazelnut Butter (1 tbsp):
Potassium: 28mg
Phosphorus: 33mg
Sodium: 0mg

Pecan Butter (1 tbsp):
Potassium: 25mg
Phosphorus: 13mg
Sodium: 0mg

Walnut Butter (1 tbsp):
Potassium: 29mg
Phosphorus: 27mg
Sodium: 0mg

Brazil Nut Butter (1 tbsp):
Potassium: 15mg
Phosphorus: 15mg
Sodium: 0mg

Macadamia Nut Butter (1 tbsp):
Potassium: 16mg
Phosphorus: 8mg
Sodium: 0mg

Sesame Seed Butter (1 tbsp):
Potassium: 52mg
Phosphorus: 60mg
Sodium: 1mg

Poppy Seed Butter (1 tbsp):
Potassium: 37mg
Phosphorus: 44mg
Sodium: 1mg

Sunflower Seed Butter (1 tbsp):
Potassium: 20mg
Phosphorus: 21mg
Sodium: 0mg

Tahini (1 tbsp):
Potassium: 79mg
Phosphorus: 37mg
Sodium: 1mg

Hemp Seed Butter (1 tbsp):
Potassium: 26mg
Phosphorus: 50mg

Sodium: 0mg

Pumpkin Seed Butter (1 tbsp):
Potassium: 41mg
Phosphorus: 44mg
Sodium: 1mg

Sunflower Seed Butter (1 tbsp):
Potassium: 39mg
Phosphorus: 42mg
Sodium: 1mg

Sunflower Seed Spread (1 tbsp):
Potassium: 22mg
Phosphorus: 23mg
Sodium: 0mg

Mixed Nut Butter (1 tbsp):
Potassium: Varies
Phosphorus: Varies
Sodium: Varies

Spices and Herbs

Basil (1 tbsp, fresh):
Potassium: 8mg
Phosphorus: 3mg
Sodium: 0mg

Parsley (1 tbsp, fresh):
Potassium: 20mg
Phosphorus: 3mg
Sodium: 1mg

Cilantro (1 tbsp, fresh):
Potassium: 11mg
Phosphorus: 2mg
Sodium: 1mg

Dill (1 tbsp, fresh):
Potassium: 12mg
Phosphorus: 3mg
Sodium: 1mg

Rosemary (1 tbsp, fresh):
Potassium: 10mg
Phosphorus: 2mg
Sodium: 0mg

Thyme (1 tbsp, fresh):
Potassium: 4mg
Phosphorus: 3mg
Sodium: 0mg

Sage (1 tbsp, fresh):
Potassium: 10mg

Phosphorus: 4mg
Sodium: 0mg

Oregano (1 tbsp, fresh):
Potassium: 15mg
Phosphorus: 5mg
Sodium: 0mg

Chives (1 tbsp, fresh):
Potassium: 11mg
Phosphorus: 3mg
Sodium: 1mg

Mint (1 tbsp, fresh):
Potassium: 4mg
Phosphorus: 1mg
Sodium: 1mg

Bay Leaf (1 leaf, dried):
Potassium: 4mg
Phosphorus: 1mg
Sodium: 1mg

Cloves (1 tsp, ground):
Potassium: 30mg
Phosphorus: 13mg
Sodium: 2mg

Cinnamon (1 tsp, ground):
Potassium: 26mg
Phosphorus: 2mg
Sodium: 0mg

Ginger (1 tsp, ground):
Potassium: 26mg
Phosphorus: 2mg
Sodium: 1mg

Nutmeg (1 tsp, ground):
Potassium: 34mg
Phosphorus: 3mg
Sodium: 0mg

Turmeric (1 tsp, ground):
Potassium: 17mg
Phosphorus: 3mg
Sodium: 1mg

Black Pepper (1 tsp, ground):
Potassium: 19mg
Phosphorus: 4mg
Sodium: 1mg

Paprika (1 tsp, ground):
Potassium: 17mg
Phosphorus: 2mg
Sodium: 1mg

Cayenne Pepper (1 tsp, ground):
Potassium: 15mg
Phosphorus: 3mg
Sodium: 1mg

Garlic Powder (1 tsp):
Potassium: 10mg

Phosphorus: 3mg
Sodium: 1mg

Onion Powder (1 tsp):
Potassium: 11mg
Phosphorus: 3mg
Sodium: 1mg

Celery Seed (1 tsp):
Potassium: 14mg
Phosphorus: 4mg
Sodium: 9mg

Mustard Seed (1 tsp):
Potassium: 20mg
Phosphorus: 17mg
Sodium: 0mg

Coriander (1 tsp, ground):
Potassium: 20mg
Phosphorus: 6mg
Sodium: 1mg

Cardamom (1 tsp, ground):
Potassium: 15mg
Phosphorus: 3mg
Sodium: 0mg

Fennel Seed (1 tsp):
Potassium: 10mg
Phosphorus: 5mg
Sodium: 1mg

Caraway Seed (1 tsp):
Potassium: 6mg
Phosphorus: 5mg
Sodium: 1mg

Anise Seed (1 tsp):
Potassium: 17mg
Phosphorus: 10mg
Sodium: 1mg

Curry Powder (1 tsp):
Potassium: 16mg
Phosphorus: 5mg
Sodium: 1mg

Chili Powder (1 tsp):
Potassium: 25mg
Phosphorus: 3mg
Sodium: 1mg

Basil (1 tsp, dried):
Potassium: 10mg
Phosphorus: 4mg
Sodium: 1mg

Parsley (1 tsp, dried):
Potassium: 6mg
Phosphorus: 1mg
Sodium: 1mg

Cilantro (1 tsp, dried):
Potassium: 6mg

Phosphorus: 1mg
Sodium: 1mg

Dill (1 tsp, dried):
Potassium: 3mg
Phosphorus: 2mg
Sodium: 1mg

Rosemary (1 tsp, dried):
Potassium: 8mg
Phosphorus: 3mg
Sodium: 1mg

Thyme (1 tsp, dried):
Potassium: 6mg
Phosphorus: 3mg
Sodium: 0mg

Sage (1 tsp, dried):
Potassium: 6mg
Phosphorus: 2mg
Sodium: 0mg

Oregano (1 tsp, dried):
Potassium: 11mg
Phosphorus: 5mg
Sodium: 1mg

Chives (1 tsp, dried):
Potassium: 8mg
Phosphorus: 1mg
Sodium: 0mg

Mint (1 tsp, dried):
Potassium: 7mg
Phosphorus: 1mg
Sodium: 0mg

Bay Leaf (1 leaf, dried):
Potassium: 4mg
Phosphorus: 1mg
Sodium: 0mg

Cloves (1 tsp, whole):
Potassium: 11mg
Phosphorus: 5mg
Sodium: 1mg

Cinnamon Stick (1 inch):
Potassium: 1mg
Phosphorus: 1mg
Sodium: 0mg

Ginger (1 tsp, dried):
Potassium: 43mg
Phosphorus: 5mg
Sodium: 2mg

Nutmeg (1 tsp, ground):
Potassium: 34mg
Phosphorus: 3mg
Sodium: 0mg

Turmeric (1 tsp, ground):
Potassium: 17mg

Phosphorus: 3mg
Sodium: 1mg

Black Pepper (1 tsp, ground):
Potassium: 19mg
Phosphorus: 4mg
Sodium: 1mg

Paprika (1 tsp, ground):
Potassium: 17mg
Phosphorus: 2mg
Sodium: 1mg

Cayenne Pepper (1 tsp, ground):
Potassium: 15mg
Phosphorus: 3mg
Sodium: 1mg

Garlic Powder (1 tsp):
Potassium: 10mg
Phosphorus: 3mg
Sodium: 1mg

Spinach (1 cup, cooked):
Potassium: 839mg
Phosphorus: 167mg
Sodium: 114mg

Kale (1 cup, cooked):
Potassium: 296mg
Phosphorus: 94mg
Sodium: 23mg
Broccoli (1 cup, cooked):
Potassium: 457mg
Phosphorus: 89mg
Sodium: 35mg

Cauliflower (1 cup, cooked):
Potassium: 176mg
Phosphorus: 40mg
Sodium: 19mg

Brussels Sprouts (1 cup, cooked):
Potassium: 342mg
Phosphorus: 69mg
Sodium: 23mg

Green Beans (1 cup, cooked):
Potassium: 211mg
Phosphorus: 38mg
Sodium: 6mg

Asparagus (1 cup, cooked):
Potassium: 288mg
Phosphorus: 73mg

Sodium: 4mg

Bell Peppers (1 cup, raw):
Potassium: 261mg
Phosphorus: 23mg
Sodium: 4mg

Cabbage (1 cup, cooked):
Potassium: 170mg
Phosphorus: 32mg
Sodium: 18mg

Carrots (1 cup, cooked):
Potassium: 352mg
Phosphorus: 43mg
Sodium: 88mg

Sweet Potatoes (1 cup, cooked):
Potassium: 542mg
Phosphorus: 61mg
Sodium: 16mg

White Potatoes (1 cup, cooked):
Potassium: 941mg
Phosphorus: 121mg
Sodium: 15mg

Squash (1 cup, cooked):
Potassium: 345mg
Phosphorus: 51mg
Sodium: 6mg

Zucchini (1 cup, cooked):

Potassium: 261mg
Phosphorus: 37mg
Sodium: 6mg

Eggplant (1 cup, cooked):
Potassium: 245mg
Phosphorus: 28mg
Sodium: 3mg

Tomatoes (1 cup, raw):
Potassium: 427mg
Phosphorus: 43mg
Sodium: 9mg

Onions (1 cup, raw):
Potassium: 233mg
Phosphorus: 38mg
Sodium: 8mg

Garlic (1 clove, raw):
Potassium: 12mg
Phosphorus: 6mg
Sodium: 1mg

Celery (1 stalk, raw):
Potassium: 104mg
Phosphorus: 24mg
Sodium: 32mg

Lettuce (1 cup, shredded, raw):
Potassium: 162mg
Phosphorus: 13mg

Sodium: 11mg

Cucumber (1 cup, sliced, raw):
Potassium: 147mg
Phosphorus: 21mg
Sodium: 2mg

Radishes (1 cup, sliced, raw):
Potassium: 270mg
Phosphorus: 36mg
Sodium: 39mg

Beets (1 cup, cooked):
Potassium: 518mg
Phosphorus: 88mg
Sodium: 106mg

Turnips (1 cup, cooked):
Potassium: 401mg
Phosphorus: 51mg
Sodium: 17mg

Parsnips (1 cup, cooked):
Potassium: 573mg
Phosphorus: 94mg
Sodium: 14mg

Radicchio (1 cup, shredded, raw):
Potassium: 218mg
Phosphorus: 32mg
Sodium: 22mg

Arugula (1 cup, raw):

Potassium: 74mg
Phosphorus: 10mg
Sodium: 6mg

Watercress (1 cup, raw):
Potassium: 112mg
Phosphorus: 17mg
Sodium: 7mg

Swiss Chard (1 cup, cooked):
Potassium: 960mg
Phosphorus: 36mg
Sodium: 313mg

Bok Choy (1 cup, cooked):
Potassium: 631mg
Phosphorus: 37mg
Sodium: 33mg

Artichokes (1 medium, cooked):
Potassium: 343mg
Phosphorus: 54mg
Sodium: 91mg

Leeks (1 cup, sliced, cooked):
Potassium: 247mg
Phosphorus: 35mg
Sodium: 15mg

Fennel (1 cup, sliced, raw):
Potassium: 360mg
Phosphorus: 50mg

Sodium: 45mg

Okra (1 cup, cooked):
Potassium: 252mg
Phosphorus: 82mg
Sodium: 8mg

Snow Peas (1 cup, raw):
Potassium: 98mg
Phosphorus: 36mg
Sodium: 3mg

Snap Peas (1 cup, raw):
Potassium: 137mg
Phosphorus: 51mg
Sodium: 2mg

Spaghetti Squash (1 cup, cooked):
Potassium: 162mg
Phosphorus: 29mg
Sodium: 17mg

Acorn Squash (1 cup, cooked):
Potassium: 896mg
Phosphorus: 68mg
Sodium: 4mg

Butternut Squash (1 cup, cooked):
Potassium: 582mg
Phosphorus: 89mg
Sodium: 8mg

Hubbard Squash (1 cup, cooked):

Potassium: 896mg
Phosphorus: 68mg
Sodium: 4mg

Pumpkin (1 cup, cooked):
Potassium: 564mg
Phosphorus: 37mg
Sodium: 2mg

Yellow Squash (1 cup, cooked):
Potassium: 197mg
Phosphorus: 33mg
Sodium: 4mg

Green Peas (1 cup, cooked):
Potassium: 180mg
Phosphorus: 108mg
Sodium: 4mg

Lima Beans (1 cup, cooked):
Potassium: 955mg
Phosphorus: 209mg
Sodium: 4mg

Kidney Beans (1 cup, cooked):
Potassium: 358mg
Phosphorus: 278mg
Sodium: 2mg

Black Beans (1 cup, cooked):
Potassium: 611mg
Phosphorus: 241mg

Sodium: 1mg

Chickpeas (1 cup, cooked):
Potassium: 477mg
Phosphorus: 80mg
Sodium: 12mg

Green Lentils (1 cup, cooked):
Potassium: 731mg
Phosphorus: 180mg
Sodium: 2mg

Red Lentils (1 cup, cooked):
Potassium: 747mg
Phosphorus: 356mg
Sodium: 2mg

Split Peas (1 cup, cooked):
Potassium: 710mg
Phosphorus: 182mg
Sodium: 3mg

Part 5

Healthy and Delicious Renal friendly recipes for CKD

Soup and stew

1. Chicken and Vegetable Soup

Ingredients:
1 lb chicken breast, diced
4 cups low-sodium chicken broth
2 carrots, sliced
2 celery stalks, diced
1 onion, chopped
2 cloves garlic, minced
1 tsp dried thyme
Salt and pepper to taste

Preparation:
In a large pot, heat some olive oil over medium heat.
Add the diced chicken breast and cook until browned.
Add the chopped onion and minced garlic, cook until softened.
Pour in the chicken broth and bring to a simmer.
Add carrots, celery, dried thyme, salt, and pepper. Let simmer for about 20 minutes or until vegetables are tender.
Adjust seasoning to taste and serve hot.

Nutritional Information:
Serving Size: 1 cup
Calories: 150
Protein: 20g
Carbohydrates: 6g
Fat: 5g
Sodium: 180mg

2. Lentil and Vegetable Stew

Ingredients:
1 cup dried lentils, rinsed
4 cups low-sodium vegetable broth
2 carrots, diced
2 celery stalks, diced
1 onion, chopped
2 cloves garlic, minced
1 tsp cumin
1 tsp paprika
Salt and pepper to taste

Preparation:
In a large pot, combine lentils, vegetable broth, carrots, celery, onion, and garlic.
Bring to a boil over high heat, then reduce heat to low and simmer for about 30 minutes or until lentils are tender.
Stir in cumin, paprika, salt, and pepper. Simmer for an additional 10 minutes.
Adjust seasoning to taste and serve hot.

Nutritional Information:
Serving Size: 1 cup
Calories: 220
Protein: 15g
Carbohydrates: 40g
Fat: 1g
Sodium: 140mg

3. Creamy Potato and Leek Soup

Ingredients:
2 leeks, chopped
4 potatoes, peeled and diced
4 cups low-sodium chicken or vegetable broth
1 cup low-fat milk
2 tbsp olive oil
Salt and pepper to taste

Preparation:
In a large pot, heat olive oil over medium heat. Add chopped leeks and cook until softened.
Add diced potatoes and chicken or vegetable broth. Bring to a boil, then reduce heat and simmer until potatoes are tender.
Use an immersion blender to blend the soup until smooth. Alternatively, transfer the soup to a blender in batches and blend until smooth.
Stir in low-fat milk and heat through.
Season with salt and pepper to taste and serve hot.

Nutritional Information:
Serving Size: 1 cup
Calories: 180
Protein: 5g
Carbohydrates: 30g
Fat: 4g
Sodium: 220mg

4. Turkey and Rice Soup

Ingredients:
1 lb ground turkey
1 cup cooked rice
4 cups low-sodium chicken broth
2 carrots, sliced
2 celery stalks, diced
1 onion, chopped
2 cloves garlic, minced
1 tsp dried thyme
Salt and pepper to taste

Preparation:
In a large pot, cook ground turkey over medium heat until browned.
Add chopped onion and minced garlic, cook until softened.
Pour in chicken broth and bring to a simmer.
Add carrots, celery, cooked rice, dried thyme, salt, and pepper. Let simmer for about 20 minutes or until vegetables are tender.
Adjust seasoning to taste and serve hot.

Nutritional Information:
Serving Size: 1 cup
Calories: 200
Protein: 15g
Carbohydrates: 20g
Fat: 7g
Sodium: 180mg

5. Minestrone Soup

Ingredients:
1 cup cooked small pasta (such as ditalini or small shells)
4 cups low-sodium vegetable broth
1 can (15 oz) kidney beans, drained and rinsed
2 carrots, diced
2 celery stalks, diced
1 onion, chopped
2 cloves garlic, minced
1 can (14.5 oz) diced tomatoes
1 tsp dried basil
1 tsp dried oregano
Salt and pepper to taste

Preparation:
In a large pot, heat some olive oil over medium heat. Add chopped onion and minced garlic, cook until softened.
Add diced carrots and celery, cook until slightly softened.
Pour in vegetable broth and bring to a simmer.

Add diced tomatoes, cooked pasta, kidney beans, dried basil, dried oregano, salt, and pepper. Let simmer for about 15-20 minutes.
Adjust seasoning to taste and serve hot.

Nutritional Information:
Serving Size: 1 cup
Calories: 180
Protein: 8g
Carbohydrates: 32g
Fat: 1g
Sodium: 220mg

Side dishes

1. Garlic Roasted Asparagus
Ingredients:

1 pound fresh asparagus spears
2 tablespoons olive oil
3 cloves garlic, minced
Salt and pepper to taste

Preparation:
Preheat oven to 400°F (200°C).
Wash and trim the tough ends of the asparagus spears.
Place the asparagus spears on a baking sheet.
In a small bowl, mix olive oil and minced garlic. Drizzle the mixture over the asparagus and toss to coat evenly.
Sprinkle with salt and pepper.
Roast in the preheated oven for 12-15 minutes, or until the asparagus is tender and slightly crispy.
Serve hot.

Nutritional Information: (Per serving)
Calories: 78 kcal
Protein: 2g
Fat: 7g
Carbohydrates: 4g
Fiber: 2g
Potassium: 234mg
Phosphorus: 46mg
Sodium: 2mg

2. Lemon Herb Quinoa

Ingredients:
1 cup quinoa, rinsed
2 cups low-sodium vegetable broth
Zest and juice of 1 lemon
2 tablespoons chopped fresh parsley
1 tablespoon chopped fresh dill
Salt and pepper to taste

Preparation:
In a saucepan, combine quinoa and vegetable broth. Bring to a boil.
Reduce heat, cover, and simmer for 15-20 minutes, or until quinoa is cooked and liquid is absorbed.
Fluff the quinoa with a fork and transfer to a serving bowl.
Stir in lemon zest, lemon juice, parsley, and dill.
Season with salt and pepper to taste.
Serve warm.

Nutritional Information: (Per serving)
Calories: 160 kcal
Protein: 6g
Fat: 2g
Carbohydrates: 31g
Fiber: 3g
Potassium: 159mg
Phosphorus: 111mg
Sodium: 22mg

3. Balsamic Glazed Carrots

Ingredients:
1 pound carrots, peeled and sliced into sticks
2 tablespoons balsamic vinegar
1 tablespoon olive oil
1 tablespoon honey
Salt and pepper to taste
Chopped fresh parsley for garnish (optional)

Preparation:
Preheat oven to 400°F (200°C).
In a bowl, whisk together balsamic vinegar, olive oil, honey, salt, and pepper.
Add the carrot sticks to the bowl and toss to coat evenly.
Spread the carrots in a single layer on a baking sheet lined with parchment paper.
Roast in the preheated oven for 20-25 minutes, or until the carrots are tender and caramelized, stirring halfway through.
Transfer the roasted carrots to a serving dish, garnish with chopped parsley if desired, and serve.

Nutritional Information: (Per serving)
Calories: 110 kcal
Protein: 1g
Fat: 3g
Carbohydrates: 20g
Fiber: 4g
Potassium: 376mg
Phosphorus: 54mg
Sodium: 71mg

4. Herb Roasted Potatoes

Ingredients:
1 pound small red potatoes, halved or quartered
2 tablespoons olive oil
1 tablespoon chopped fresh rosemary
1 tablespoon chopped fresh thyme
Salt and pepper to taste

Preparation:
Preheat oven to 400°F (200°C).
In a bowl, toss the potato halves with olive oil, chopped rosemary, chopped thyme, salt, and pepper until evenly coated.
Spread the potatoes in a single layer on a baking sheet lined with parchment paper.
Roast in the preheated oven for 25-30 minutes, or until the potatoes are golden brown and tender, stirring halfway through.
Serve hot.

Nutritional Information: (Per serving)
Calories: 132 kcal
Protein: 2g
Fat: 7g
Carbohydrates: 16g
Fiber: 2g
Potassium: 356mg
Phosphorus: 51mg
Sodium: 7mg

5. Lemon Garlic Green Beans

Ingredients:
1 pound fresh green beans, trimmed
2 tablespoons olive oil
2 cloves garlic, minced
Zest and juice of 1 lemon
Salt and pepper to taste

Preparation:
Bring a large pot of salted water to a boil. Add green beans and blanch for 2-3 minutes, until bright green and slightly tender. Drain and rinse under cold water to stop cooking.
In a large skillet, heat olive oil over medium heat. Add minced garlic and sauté for 1-2 minutes until fragrant.
Add blanched green beans to the skillet. Cook, stirring occasionally, for 2-3 minutes until heated through.
Stir in lemon zest and lemon juice. Season with salt and pepper to taste.
Transfer to a serving dish and serve immediately.

Nutritional Information: (Per serving)
Calories: 84 kcal
Protein: 2g
Fat: 5g
Carbohydrates: 10g
Fiber: 4g
Potassium: 244mg
Phosphorus: 46mg
Sodium: 6mg

Mains

1. Lemon Herb Grilled Chicken Breast

Ingredients:
4 boneless, skinless chicken breasts
2 tablespoons olive oil
Zest and juice of 1 lemon
2 cloves garlic, minced
1 tablespoon chopped fresh parsley
1 tablespoon chopped fresh thyme
Salt and pepper to taste

Preparation:
In a bowl, whisk together olive oil, lemon zest, lemon juice, minced garlic, chopped parsley, chopped thyme, salt, and pepper to create a marinade.
Place the chicken breasts in a shallow dish and pour the marinade over them. Ensure the chicken is evenly coated. Marinate in the refrigerator for at least 30 minutes.
Preheat grill to medium-high heat. Remove chicken from marinade and discard excess marinade.

Grill chicken breasts for 6-8 minutes per side, or until cooked through and no longer pink in the center.
Remove from grill and let rest for a few minutes before serving.

Nutritional Information: (Per serving)
Calories: 220 kcal
Protein: 26g
Fat: 11g
Carbohydrates: 3g
Fiber: 1g
Potassium: 304mg
Phosphorus: 213mg
Sodium: 85mg

2. Baked Salmon with Dill Sauce

Ingredients:
4 salmon fillets (about 6 ounces each)
2 tablespoons olive oil
Salt and pepper to taste
1 tablespoon chopped fresh dill
1 tablespoon lemon juice
1/2 cup plain Greek yogurt
1 clove garlic, minced

Preparation:
Preheat oven to 400°F (200°C). Line a baking sheet with parchment paper.
Place the salmon fillets on the prepared baking sheet. Drizzle with olive oil and season with salt and pepper.
Bake for 12-15 minutes, or until the salmon is cooked through and flakes easily with a fork.

While the salmon is baking, prepare the dill sauce. In a small bowl, mix together chopped dill, lemon juice, Greek yogurt, minced garlic, salt, and pepper.
Serve the baked salmon hot with a dollop of dill sauce on top.

Nutritional Information: (Per serving)
Calories: 340 kcal
Protein: 34g
Fat: 20g
Carbohydrates: 3g
Fiber: 0g
Potassium: 706mg
Phosphorus: 445mg
Sodium: 117mg

3. Turkey and Vegetable Stir-Fry

Ingredients:
1 pound turkey breast, thinly sliced
2 tablespoons olive oil
2 cups mixed vegetables (such as bell peppers, broccoli, carrots, and snow peas)
2 cloves garlic, minced
2 tablespoons low-sodium soy sauce
1 tablespoon rice vinegar
1 teaspoon honey
1 teaspoon cornstarch (optional, for thickening)
Cooked brown rice or quinoa for serving

Preparation:
Heat olive oil in a large skillet or wok over medium-high heat. Add minced garlic and sauté for 1 minute until fragrant.
Add sliced turkey breast to the skillet and stir-fry until browned and cooked through.
Add mixed vegetables to the skillet and continue to stir-fry for 3-4 minutes, or until vegetables are tender-crisp.
In a small bowl, whisk together low-sodium soy sauce, rice vinegar, honey, and cornstarch (if using).
Pour the sauce over the turkey and vegetables in the skillet. Stir well to coat evenly and allow the sauce to thicken slightly.
Serve the turkey and vegetable stir-fry hot over cooked brown rice or quinoa.

Nutritional Information: (Per serving, excluding rice/quinoa)
Calories: 250 kcal
Protein: 26g
Fat: 10g
Carbohydrates: 14g
Fiber: 3g
Potassium: 412mg
Phosphorus: 294mg
Sodium: 357mg

4. Eggplant Parmesan

Ingredients:
1 large eggplant, sliced into rounds
2 eggs, beaten
1 cup breadcrumbs (preferably whole wheat)

1/4 cup grated Parmesan cheese
2 cups low-sodium marinara sauce
1 cup shredded mozzarella cheese
Fresh basil leaves for garnish (optional)

Preparation:
Preheat oven to 375°F (190°C). Line a baking sheet with parchment paper.
Dip eggplant slices into beaten eggs, then coat them in a mixture of breadcrumbs and grated Parmesan cheese.
Place the coated eggplant slices on the prepared baking sheet in a single layer.
Bake in the preheated oven for 20-25 minutes, or until the eggplant is tender and golden brown.
Remove the eggplant slices from the oven and increase the oven temperature to 400°F (200°C).
In a baking dish, spread a thin layer of marinara sauce. Arrange half of the baked eggplant slices on top of the sauce.
Top the eggplant slices with more marinara sauce and shredded mozzarella cheese. Repeat with another layer of eggplant slices, sauce, and cheese.
Bake in the oven for an additional 15-20 minutes, or until the cheese is melted and bubbly.
Garnish with fresh basil leaves before serving.

Nutritional Information: (Per serving)
Calories: 290 kcal
Protein: 16g
Fat: 12g
Carbohydrates: 30g
Fiber: 6g
Potassium: 606mg

Phosphorus: 268mg
Sodium: 482mg

5. Vegetable and Tofu Stir-Fry

Ingredients:
1 block firm tofu, pressed and cubed
2 tablespoons olive oil
2 cups mixed vegetables (such as bell peppers, broccoli, carrots, and snap peas)
2 cloves garlic, minced
2 tablespoons low-sodium soy sauce
1 tablespoon hoisin sauce
1 tablespoon rice vinegar
1 teaspoon sesame oil
Cooked brown rice or quinoa for serving

Preparation:
Heat olive oil in a large skillet or wok over medium-high heat. Add minced garlic and sauté for 1 minute until fragrant.
Add cubed tofu to the skillet and stir-fry until lightly golden brown on all sides.
Add mixed vegetables to the skillet and continue to stir-fry for 3-4 minutes, or until vegetables are tender-crisp.
In a small bowl, whisk together low-sodium soy sauce, hoisin sauce, rice vinegar, and sesame oil.
Pour the sauce over the tofu and vegetables in the skillet. Stir well to coat evenly.
Cook for an additional 1-2 minutes until the sauce has thickened slightly.
Serve the vegetable and tofu stir-fry hot over cooked brown rice or quinoa.

Nutritional Information: (Per serving, excluding rice/quinoa)
Calories: 290 kcal
Protein: 16g
Fat: 18g
Carbohydrates: 20g
Fiber: 5g
Potassium: 538mg
Phosphorus: 249mg
Sodium: 396mg

Salads

1. Greek Salad

Ingredients:
2 cups chopped romaine lettuce
1 cucumber, sliced
1 cup cherry tomatoes, halved
1/2 red onion, thinly sliced
1/4 cup crumbled feta cheese
2 tablespoons Kalamata olives, pitted
2 tablespoons olive oil
1 tablespoon red wine vinegar
1 teaspoon dried oregano
Salt and pepper to taste

Preparation:
In a large salad bowl, combine chopped romaine lettuce, sliced cucumber, halved cherry tomatoes, thinly sliced red onion, crumbled feta cheese, and pitted Kalamata olives.

In a small bowl, whisk together olive oil, red wine vinegar, dried oregano, salt, and pepper to make the dressing.
Pour the dressing over the salad ingredients and toss gently to coat.
Serve immediately as a refreshing side dish or light meal.

Nutritional Information: (Per serving)
Calories: 130 kcal
Protein: 3g
Fat: 10g
Carbohydrates: 8g
Fiber: 2g
Potassium: 312mg
Phosphorus: 62mg
Sodium: 201mg

2. Spinach and Strawberry Salad

Ingredients:
3 cups baby spinach leaves
1 cup sliced strawberries
1/4 cup chopped walnuts
2 tablespoons crumbled goat cheese
2 tablespoons balsamic vinegar
1 tablespoon olive oil
1 teaspoon honey
Salt and pepper to taste

Preparation:
In a large salad bowl, combine baby spinach leaves, sliced strawberries, chopped walnuts, and crumbled goat cheese.
In a small bowl, whisk together balsamic vinegar, olive oil, honey, salt, and pepper to make the dressing.
Drizzle the dressing over the salad ingredients and toss gently to coat.
Serve immediately as a vibrant and flavorful salad.

Nutritional Information: (Per serving)
Calories: 180 kcal
Protein: 4g
Fat: 13g
Carbohydrates: 14g
Fiber: 3g
Potassium: 378mg
Phosphorus: 94mg
Sodium: 69mg

3. Avocado and Tomato Salad

Ingredients:
2 ripe avocados, diced
1 cup cherry tomatoes, halved
1/4 red onion, thinly sliced
1/4 cup chopped fresh cilantro
Juice of 1 lime
2 tablespoons olive oil
Salt and pepper to taste

Preparation:
In a large salad bowl, combine diced avocados, halved cherry tomatoes, thinly sliced red onion, and chopped fresh cilantro.
Drizzle lime juice and olive oil over the salad ingredients.
Season with salt and pepper to taste.
Toss gently to coat everything evenly.
Serve immediately as a creamy and refreshing salad.

Nutritional Information: (Per serving)
Calories: 210 kcal
Protein: 3g
Fat: 19g
Carbohydrates: 11g
Fiber: 7g
Potassium: 630mg
Phosphorus: 89mg
Sodium: 11mg

4. Quinoa and Black Bean Salad

Ingredients:
1 cup cooked quinoa, cooled
1 can (15 ounces) black beans, rinsed and drained
1 cup diced bell peppers (any color)
1/2 cup diced red onion
1/4 cup chopped fresh cilantro
Juice of 1 lime
2 tablespoons olive oil
1 teaspoon ground cumin
Salt and pepper to taste

Preparation:
In a large salad bowl, combine cooked quinoa, black beans, diced bell peppers, diced red onion, and chopped fresh cilantro.
In a small bowl, whisk together lime juice, olive oil, ground cumin, salt, and pepper to make the dressing.
Pour the dressing over the salad ingredients and toss gently to coat.
Serve immediately as a protein-packed and nutritious salad.

Nutritional Information: (Per serving)
Calories: 250 kcal
Protein: 9g
Fat: 8g
Carbohydrates: 38g
Fiber: 9g
Potassium: 491mg
Phosphorus: 159mg
Sodium: 259mg

5. Tuna and White Bean Salad

Ingredients:
1 can (15 ounces) white beans (such as cannellini or Great Northern), rinsed and drained
1 can (5 ounces) tuna in water, drained and flaked
1/2 cup diced celery
1/4 cup chopped red onion
2 tablespoons chopped fresh parsley
Juice of 1 lemon
2 tablespoons olive oil
Salt and pepper to taste

Preparation:
In a large salad bowl, combine white beans, flaked tuna, diced celery, chopped red onion, and chopped fresh parsley.
Drizzle lemon juice and olive oil over the salad ingredients.
Season with salt and pepper to taste.
Toss gently to combine everything evenly.
Serve immediately as a protein-rich and satisfying salad.

Nutritional Information: (Per serving)
Calories: 290 kcal
Protein: 23g
Fat: 10g
Carbohydrates: 28g
Fiber: 7g
Potassium: 650mg
Phosphorus: 244mg
Sodium: 363mg

Snack and Appetizer

1. Hummus with Fresh Vegetables

Ingredients:
1 can (15 ounces) chickpeas, drained and rinsed
2 tablespoons tahini
2 cloves garlic, minced
Juice of 1 lemon
2 tablespoons olive oil
Salt and pepper to taste

Assorted fresh vegetables for dipping (carrots, cucumber, bell peppers, etc.)

Preparation:
In a food processor, combine chickpeas, tahini, minced garlic, lemon juice, olive oil, salt, and pepper.
Blend until smooth and creamy, adding a little water if needed to reach desired consistency.
Transfer the hummus to a serving bowl.
Wash and prepare the fresh vegetables for dipping.
Serve the hummus with the assorted fresh vegetables for a healthy and satisfying snack.

Nutritional Information: (Per serving, excluding vegetables)
Calories: 130 kcal
Protein: 5g
Fat: 7g
Carbohydrates: 13g
Fiber: 4g
Potassium: 185mg
Phosphorus: 86mg
Sodium: 94mg

2. Stuffed Cucumber Bites

Ingredients:
2 large cucumbers
1/2 cup low-fat cream cheese
1/4 cup chopped fresh dill
1 tablespoon lemon juice
Salt and pepper to taste
Cherry tomatoes for garnish

Preparation:
Peel the cucumbers and slice them into rounds, about 1/2 inch thick.
Use a small spoon or melon baller to scoop out the seeds from the center of each cucumber round, creating a hollow space.
In a bowl, mix together low-fat cream cheese, chopped fresh dill, lemon juice, salt, and pepper.
Spoon the cream cheese mixture into the hollowed-out cucumber rounds.
Garnish each stuffed cucumber bite with a cherry tomato on top.
Arrange the stuffed cucumber bites on a serving platter and serve chilled.

Nutritional Information: (Per serving)
Calories: 35 kcal
Protein: 2g
Fat: 2g
Carbohydrates: 3g
Fiber: 1g
Potassium: 160mg
Phosphorus: 34mg
Sodium: 35mg

3. Roasted Chickpeas

Ingredients:
1 can (15 ounces) chickpeas, drained and rinsed
1 tablespoon olive oil
1 teaspoon paprika
1/2 teaspoon garlic powder
1/2 teaspoon cumin

Salt to taste

Preparation:
Preheat oven to 400°F (200°C). Line a baking sheet with parchment paper.
Pat the chickpeas dry with a paper towel to remove excess moisture.
In a bowl, toss the chickpeas with olive oil, paprika, garlic powder, cumin, and salt until evenly coated.
Spread the seasoned chickpeas in a single layer on the prepared baking sheet.
Roast in the preheated oven for 25-30 minutes, stirring halfway through, until crispy and golden brown.
Remove from the oven and let cool before serving as a crunchy and flavorful snack.

Nutritional Information: (Per serving)
Calories: 130 kcal
Protein: 5g
Fat: 4g
Carbohydrates: 18g
Fiber: 5g
Potassium: 200mg
Phosphorus: 80mg
Sodium: 160mg

4. Caprese Skewers

Ingredients:
Cherry tomatoes
Fresh mozzarella balls
Fresh basil leaves
Balsamic glaze (store-bought or homemade)

Preparation:
Assemble the caprese skewers by threading one cherry tomato, one fresh mozzarella ball, and one fresh basil leaf onto small skewers or toothpicks.
Arrange the assembled skewers on a serving platter.
Drizzle balsamic glaze over the skewers just before serving.
Serve immediately as a simple and elegant appetizer.

Nutritional Information: (Per serving)
Calories: 45 kcal
Protein: 3g
Fat: 3g
Carbohydrates: 2g
Fiber: 0g
Potassium: 40mg
Phosphorus: 60mg
Sodium: 20mg

5. Baked Zucchini Chips

Ingredients:
2 medium zucchini, thinly sliced
1 tablespoon olive oil
1/4 cup grated Parmesan cheese
1/2 teaspoon garlic powder
Salt and pepper to taste

Preparation:
Preheat oven to 425°F (220°C). Line a baking sheet with parchment paper.
In a bowl, toss the thinly sliced zucchini with olive oil, grated Parmesan cheese, garlic powder, salt, and pepper until evenly coated.
Arrange the seasoned zucchini slices in a single layer on the prepared baking sheet.
Bake in the preheated oven for 15-20 minutes, flipping halfway through, until the zucchini chips are golden brown and crispy.
Remove from the oven and let cool before serving as a crunchy and flavorful snack.

Nutritional Information: (Per serving)
Calories: 70 kcal
Protein: 3g
Fat: 5g
Carbohydrates: 4g
Fiber: 1g
Potassium: 310mg
Phosphorus: 63mg
Sodium: 105mg

Cooking Techniques to Reduce Sodium and Phosphorus in Meals

Reducing sodium and phosphorus in meals is crucial for individuals with chronic kidney disease (CKD) as excessive intake of these minerals can exacerbate kidney damage and lead to complications. Here are some cooking techniques to help reduce sodium and phosphorus content in meals:

Cooking Techniques to Reduce Sodium:
Limit the Use of Salt: Instead of salt, use herbs, spices, and other flavorings to enhance the taste of your dishes. Experiment with fresh herbs like basil, cilantro, rosemary, and thyme, or spices such as garlic powder, onion powder, cumin, and paprika.

Rinse Canned Foods: Canned foods, including vegetables, beans, and fish, often contain high levels of sodium due to the preserving process. Rinse canned foods thoroughly under running water before using them to remove excess salt.

Choose Low-Sodium Ingredients: Opt for low-sodium or no-added-salt versions of ingredients like broth, canned tomatoes, and condiments such as soy sauce and mustard. Read food labels carefully and select products with the lowest sodium content.

Make Your Own Sauces and Dressings: Store-bought sauces and dressings can be high in sodium. Prepare homemade versions using low-sodium ingredients like vinegar, lemon juice, olive oil, and fresh herbs.

Cook from Scratch: Processed and pre-packaged foods often contain hidden sodium. Cooking meals from scratch allows you to control the sodium content and choose healthier ingredients.

Cooking Techniques to Reduce Phosphorus:
Choose Low-Phosphorus Ingredients: Select foods that are naturally low in phosphorus, such as fresh fruits and vegetables, lean meats, poultry, and fish. Avoid processed and packaged foods that may contain phosphate additives.

Soak and Boil Beans: Beans and legumes are high in phosphorus, but soaking them in water overnight and boiling them in fresh water can help reduce their phosphorus content. Drain and rinse the beans thoroughly after soaking.

Trim Meat and Poultry: Trim visible fat from meat and poultry before cooking to reduce phosphorus intake. Opt for lean cuts of meat and remove skin from poultry.

Use Dairy Alternatives: Dairy products like milk, cheese, and yogurt are significant sources of phosphorus. Choose dairy alternatives such as almond milk, coconut milk, or rice milk, which have lower phosphorus content.

Limit Processed Foods: Processed and convenience foods often contain phosphate additives to enhance flavor and texture. Minimize consumption of processed foods like deli meats, frozen meals, and packaged snacks.

Grill or Broil Instead of Fry: When cooking meat or fish, grill or broil them instead of frying. This method helps reduce the absorption of phosphorus from the cooking oil.

30 days kidney diseases meals plan

Day 1: Grilled Lemon Herb Chicken

Ingredients:
4 boneless, skinless chicken breasts
2 tablespoons olive oil
Zest and juice of 1 lemon
2 cloves garlic, minced
1 tablespoon chopped fresh parsley
1 tablespoon chopped fresh thyme
Salt and pepper to taste

Preparation:
In a bowl, mix together olive oil, lemon zest, lemon juice, minced garlic, chopped parsley, chopped thyme, salt, and pepper to create a marinade.
Place chicken breasts in a shallow dish and pour the marinade over them. Marinate in the refrigerator for at least 30 minutes.
Preheat grill to medium-high heat. Remove chicken from marinade and discard excess marinade.
Grill chicken breasts for 6-8 minutes per side, or until cooked through.
Let rest for a few minutes before serving.
Prep Time: 40 minutes
Recommended Potassium: 290mg
Phosphorus: 213mg
Sodium: 85mg

Day 2: Quinoa and Black Bean Salad

Ingredients:
1 cup cooked quinoa, cooled
1 can (15 ounces) black beans, rinsed and drained
1 cup diced bell peppers
1/2 cup diced red onion
1/4 cup chopped fresh cilantro
Juice of 1 lime
2 tablespoons olive oil
1 teaspoon ground cumin
Salt and pepper to taste

Preparation:
In a bowl, combine quinoa, black beans, bell peppers, red onion, cilantro, lime juice, olive oil, cumin, salt, and pepper.
Toss gently to combine.
Serve chilled or at room temperature.
Prep Time: 20 minutes
Recommended Potassium: 280mg
Phosphorus: 159mg
Sodium: 259mg

Day 3: Baked Salmon with Dill Sauce

Ingredients:
4 salmon fillets
2 tablespoons olive oil
Salt and pepper to taste
1 tablespoon chopped fresh dill
1 tablespoon lemon juice
1/2 cup plain Greek yogurt

1 clove garlic, minced

Preparation:
Preheat oven to 400°F (200°C). Line a baking sheet with parchment paper.
Place salmon fillets on prepared baking sheet. Drizzle with olive oil and season with salt and pepper.
Bake for 12-15 minutes, or until cooked through.
In a bowl, mix together dill, lemon juice, Greek yogurt, and minced garlic.
Serve salmon with dill sauce.
Prep Time: 20 minutes
Recommended Potassium: 706mg
Phosphorus: 445mg
Sodium: 117mg

Day 4: Vegetable and Tofu Stir-Fry

Ingredients:
1 block firm tofu, cubed
2 tablespoons olive oil
2 cups mixed vegetables
2 cloves garlic, minced
2 tablespoons low-sodium soy sauce
1 tablespoon hoisin sauce
1 tablespoon rice vinegar
1 teaspoon sesame oil

Preparation:
Heat olive oil in a skillet or wok over medium-high heat.
Add tofu and cook until browned.
Add mixed vegetables and garlic. Stir-fry until tender.

In a small bowl, whisk together soy sauce, hoisin sauce, rice vinegar, and sesame oil.
Pour sauce over tofu and vegetables. Cook until heated through.
Prep Time: 25 minutes
Recommended Potassium: 538mg
Phosphorus: 249mg
Sodium: 396mg

Day 5: Hummus with Fresh Vegetables

Ingredients:
1 can (15 ounces) chickpeas, drained and rinsed
2 tablespoons tahini
2 cloves garlic, minced
Juice of 1 lemon
2 tablespoons olive oil
Salt and pepper to taste
Assorted fresh vegetables for dipping

Preparation:
In a food processor, blend chickpeas, tahini, garlic, lemon juice, olive oil, salt, and pepper until smooth.
Serve hummus with fresh vegetables for dipping.
Prep Time: 15 minutes
Recommended Potassium: 185mg
Phosphorus: 86mg
Sodium: 94mg

Day 6: Eggplant Parmesan

Ingredients:
1 large eggplant, sliced

2 eggs, beaten
1 cup breadcrumbs
1/4 cup grated Parmesan cheese
2 cups low-sodium marinara sauce
1 cup shredded mozzarella cheese
Fresh basil leaves for garnish (optional)

Preparation:
Preheat oven to 375°F (190°C). Line a baking sheet with parchment paper.
Dip eggplant slices into beaten eggs, then coat with breadcrumbs mixed with grated Parmesan cheese.
Arrange coated eggplant slices on baking sheet. Bake for 20-25 minutes until tender.
In a baking dish, spread marinara sauce. Arrange baked eggplant slices on top. Top with remaining marinara sauce and mozzarella cheese.
Bake for an additional 15-20 minutes until cheese is melted and bubbly. Garnish with fresh basil leaves before serving.
Prep Time: 50 minutes
Recommended Potassium: 606mg
Phosphorus: 268mg
Sodium: 482mg

Day 7: Tuna and White Bean Salad

Ingredients:
1 can (15 ounces) white beans, rinsed and drained
1 can (5 ounces) tuna in water, drained and flaked
1/2 cup diced celery
1/4 cup chopped red onion
2 tablespoons chopped fresh parsley

Juice of 1 lemon
2 tablespoons olive oil
Salt and pepper to taste

Preparation:
In a large bowl, combine white beans, flaked tuna, diced celery, chopped red onion, and chopped parsley.
Drizzle lemon juice and olive oil over salad. Season with salt and pepper.
Toss gently to combine all ingredients.
Serve as a refreshing salad.
Prep Time: 15 minutes
Recommended Potassium: 650mg
Phosphorus: 244mg
Sodium: 363mg

Day 8: Lemon Garlic Shrimp

Ingredients:
1 pound shrimp, peeled and deveined
2 tablespoons olive oil
3 cloves garlic, minced
Zest and juice of 1 lemon
1 tablespoon chopped fresh parsley
Salt and pepper to taste

Preparation:
In a bowl, combine shrimp with olive oil, minced garlic, lemon zest, lemon juice, chopped parsley, salt, and pepper.
Marinate shrimp for 15-30 minutes.

Heat a skillet over medium-high heat. Add shrimp and cook for 2-3 minutes per side until pink and cooked through.
Serve shrimp hot with lemon wedges for garnish.
Prep Time: 20 minutes
Recommended Potassium: 370mg
Phosphorus: 181mg
Sodium: 220mg

Day 9: Caprese Salad

Ingredients:
2 large tomatoes, sliced
1 ball fresh mozzarella cheese, sliced
Fresh basil leaves
Balsamic glaze
Salt and pepper to taste

Preparation:
Arrange tomato and mozzarella slices alternately on a plate.
Tuck fresh basil leaves between slices.
Drizzle with balsamic glaze and sprinkle with salt and pepper.
Serve as a light and flavorful salad.
Prep Time: 10 minutes
Recommended Potassium: 550mg
Phosphorus: 400mg
Sodium: 300mg

Day 10: Lentil Soup

Ingredients:

1 cup dried lentils, rinsed
4 cups low-sodium chicken or vegetable broth
1 onion, diced
2 carrots, diced
2 stalks celery, diced
2 cloves garlic, minced
1 teaspoon ground cumin
1/2 teaspoon smoked paprika
Salt and pepper to taste
Chopped fresh parsley for garnish

Preparation:
In a large pot, combine lentils, broth, onion, carrots, celery, garlic, cumin, and paprika.
Bring to a boil, then reduce heat and simmer for 25-30 minutes until lentils and vegetables are tender.
Season with salt and pepper to taste.
Serve hot, garnished with chopped fresh parsley.
Prep Time: 40 minutes
Recommended Potassium: 710mg
Phosphorus: 360mg
Sodium: 210mg

Day 11: Vegetable Stir-Fry with Brown Rice

Ingredients:
2 cups mixed vegetables (such as bell peppers, broccoli, carrots, and snap peas)
1 tablespoon olive oil
2 cloves garlic, minced
2 tablespoons low-sodium soy sauce
1 tablespoon hoisin sauce
1 tablespoon rice vinegar

1 teaspoon sesame oil
Cooked brown rice for serving

Preparation:
Heat olive oil in a large skillet or wok over medium-high heat. Add minced garlic and sauté for 1 minute until fragrant.
Add mixed vegetables to the skillet and stir-fry for 3-4 minutes, or until vegetables are tender-crisp.
In a small bowl, whisk together low-sodium soy sauce, hoisin sauce, rice vinegar, and sesame oil.
Pour the sauce over the vegetables in the skillet. Stir well to coat evenly.
Cook for an additional 1-2 minutes until the sauce has thickened slightly.
Serve the vegetable stir-fry hot over cooked brown rice.
Prep Time: 20 minutes
Recommended Potassium: 350mg
Phosphorus: 98mg
Sodium: 380mg

Day 12: Chicken and Vegetable Kebabs

Ingredients:
2 boneless, skinless chicken breasts, cut into cubes
1 bell pepper, cut into chunks
1 zucchini, sliced
1 onion, cut into wedges
2 tablespoons olive oil
2 tablespoons balsamic vinegar
1 teaspoon dried oregano
Salt and pepper to taste

Preparation:
In a bowl, mix together olive oil, balsamic vinegar, dried oregano, salt, and pepper.
Thread chicken cubes, bell pepper chunks, zucchini slices, and onion wedges onto skewers.
Brush the kebabs with the prepared marinade.
Preheat grill to medium-high heat. Grill kebabs for 10-12 minutes, turning occasionally, until chicken is cooked through and vegetables are tender.
Serve hot with a side of rice or salad.
Prep Time: 30 minutes
Recommended Potassium: 490mg
Phosphorus: 250mg
Sodium: 100mg

Day 13: Cauliflower Rice Stir-Fry

Ingredients:
1 head cauliflower, grated into rice-like texture
2 tablespoons olive oil
2 cloves garlic, minced
1 cup mixed vegetables (such as carrots, peas, and corn)
2 eggs, beaten
2 tablespoons low-sodium soy sauce
1 tablespoon hoisin sauce
1 teaspoon sesame oil
Chopped green onions for garnish

Preparation:
Heat olive oil in a large skillet or wok over medium heat. Add minced garlic and sauté for 1 minute.
Add mixed vegetables and cook until tender.

Push vegetables to one side of the skillet and pour beaten eggs into the other side. Scramble until cooked through.

Add grated cauliflower to the skillet and stir-fry for 3-4 minutes until heated through.

In a small bowl, whisk together low-sodium soy sauce, hoisin sauce, and sesame oil. Pour over the cauliflower mixture and toss to combine.

Cook for an additional 2-3 minutes, then garnish with chopped green onions before serving.

Prep Time: 25 minutes
Recommended Potassium: 400mg
Phosphorus: 110mg
Sodium: 280mg

Day 14: Turkey and Vegetable Chili

Ingredients:
1 tablespoon olive oil
1 onion, diced
2 cloves garlic, minced
1 pound ground turkey
1 bell pepper, diced
1 zucchini, diced
1 can (15 ounces) diced tomatoes
1 can (15 ounces) kidney beans, drained and rinsed
1 tablespoon chili powder
1 teaspoon ground cumin
Salt and pepper to taste
Chopped fresh cilantro for garnish

Preparation:

Heat olive oil in a large pot over medium heat. Add diced onion and minced garlic. Sauté until softened.

Add ground turkey and cook until browned, breaking it apart with a spoon.

Add diced bell pepper and zucchini. Cook for a few minutes until vegetables are slightly softened.

Stir in diced tomatoes, kidney beans, chili powder, cumin, salt, and pepper.

Simmer chili for 20-25 minutes, stirring occasionally, until flavors are well combined and vegetables are tender.

Serve hot, garnished with chopped fresh cilantro.

Prep Time: 40 minutes

Recommended Potassium: 620mg

Phosphorus: 350mg

Sodium: 270mg

Day 15: Greek Yogurt Parfait

Ingredients:
1 cup plain Greek yogurt
1/2 cup mixed berries (such as strawberries, blueberries, and raspberries)
2 tablespoons chopped nuts (such as almonds or walnuts)
1 tablespoon honey (optional)

Preparation:
In a glass or bowl, layer Greek yogurt, mixed berries, and chopped nuts.
Drizzle honey over the top if desired.
Serve immediately as a healthy and satisfying snack or dessert.

Prep Time: 5 minutes
Recommended Potassium: 200mg
Phosphorus: 150mg
Sodium: 50mg

Day 16: Lemon Herb Grilled Swordfish

Ingredients:
4 swordfish steaks
2 tablespoons olive oil
Zest and juice of 1 lemon
2 cloves garlic, minced
1 tablespoon chopped fresh parsley
1 tablespoon chopped fresh thyme
Salt and pepper to taste

Preparation:
In a bowl, mix together olive oil, lemon zest, lemon juice, minced garlic, chopped parsley, chopped thyme, salt, and pepper to create a marinade.
Place swordfish steaks in a shallow dish and pour the marinade over them. Marinate in the refrigerator for at least 30 minutes.
Preheat grill to medium-high heat. Remove swordfish from marinade and discard excess marinade.
Grill swordfish steaks for 5-6 minutes per side, or until cooked through.
Let rest for a few minutes before serving.
Prep Time: 40 minutes
Recommended Potassium: 550mg
Phosphorus: 400mg
Sodium: 280mg

Day 17: Lentil and Vegetable Soup

Ingredients:
1 cup dried lentils, rinsed
4 cups low-sodium vegetable broth
1 onion, diced
2 carrots, diced
2 stalks celery, diced
2 cloves garlic, minced
1 teaspoon dried thyme
1 teaspoon dried rosemary
Salt and pepper to taste
Chopped fresh parsley for garnish

Preparation:
In a large pot, combine lentils, vegetable broth, diced onion, diced carrots, diced celery, minced garlic, dried thyme, and dried rosemary.
Bring to a boil, then reduce heat and simmer for 25-30 minutes until lentils and vegetables are tender.
Season with salt and pepper to taste.
Serve hot, garnished with chopped fresh parsley.
Prep Time: 40 minutes
Recommended Potassium: 720mg
Phosphorus: 360mg
Sodium: 210mg

Day 18: Grilled Vegetable Platter

Ingredients:
Assorted vegetables (such as bell peppers, zucchini, eggplant, mushrooms, and cherry tomatoes)
2 tablespoons olive oil

2 cloves garlic, minced
1 tablespoon chopped fresh herbs (such as rosemary, thyme, or oregano)
Salt and pepper to taste

Preparation:
Preheat grill to medium-high heat.
Cut vegetables into large chunks or slices.
In a bowl, toss vegetables with olive oil, minced garlic, chopped fresh herbs, salt, and pepper.
Grill vegetables for 5-7 minutes per side, or until tender and lightly charred.
Arrange grilled vegetables on a platter and serve hot.
Prep Time: 20 minutes
Recommended Potassium: Varies depending on vegetables
Phosphorus: Varies depending on vegetables
Sodium: Varies depending on seasoning

Day 19: Chicken and Vegetable Curry

Ingredients:
2 boneless, skinless chicken breasts, cut into cubes
1 tablespoon olive oil
1 onion, diced
2 cloves garlic, minced
1 tablespoon curry powder
1 teaspoon ground cumin
1 teaspoon ground coriander
1 can (14 ounces) coconut milk
2 cups mixed vegetables (such as bell peppers, carrots, and peas)
Salt and pepper to taste

Cooked rice for serving

Preparation:
Heat olive oil in a large skillet over medium heat. Add diced onion and minced garlic. Sauté until softened.
Add cubed chicken breast to the skillet and cook until browned.
Stir in curry powder, ground cumin, and ground coriander. Cook for 1-2 minutes until fragrant.
Pour coconut milk into the skillet and bring to a simmer. Add mixed vegetables and simmer for 10-15 minutes until vegetables are tender and chicken is cooked through.
Season with salt and pepper to taste.
Serve hot over cooked rice.
Prep Time: 30 minutes
Recommended Potassium: 520mg
Phosphorus: 280mg
Sodium: 180mg

Day 20: Mixed Berry Smoothie Bowl

Ingredients:
1 cup frozen mixed berries (such as strawberries, blueberries, and raspberries)
1 banana, sliced
1/2 cup plain Greek yogurt
1/4 cup almond milk (or any milk of choice)
1 tablespoon honey (optional)
Toppings: sliced fresh fruit, granola, chopped nuts, shredded coconut

Preparation:

In a blender, combine frozen mixed berries, sliced banana, Greek yogurt, almond milk, and honey (if using). Blend until smooth and creamy.
Pour the smoothie into a bowl.
Top with sliced fresh fruit, granola, chopped nuts, and shredded coconut.
Serve immediately and enjoy with a spoon.
Prep Time: 5 minutes
Recommended Potassium: 300mg
Phosphorus: 200mg
Sodium: 100mg

Day 21: Grilled Lemon Garlic Shrimp Skewers

Ingredients:
1 pound large shrimp, peeled and deveined
2 tablespoons olive oil
Zest and juice of 1 lemon
3 cloves garlic, minced
1 tablespoon chopped fresh parsley
Salt and pepper to taste

Preparation:
In a bowl, whisk together olive oil, lemon zest, lemon juice, minced garlic, chopped parsley, salt, and pepper.
Thread shrimp onto skewers.
Brush shrimp skewers with the prepared marinade.
Preheat grill to medium-high heat. Grill skewers for 2-3 minutes per side, or until shrimp are pink and opaque.
Serve hot with lemon wedges for squeezing.
Prep Time: 20 minutes
Recommended Potassium: 150mg
Phosphorus: 175mg

Sodium: 190mg

Day 22: Baked Cod with Herbed Breadcrumb Topping

Ingredients:
4 cod fillets
2 tablespoons olive oil
1 cup breadcrumbs
1/4 cup grated Parmesan cheese
2 cloves garlic, minced
1 tablespoon chopped fresh parsley
1 teaspoon chopped fresh thyme
Salt and pepper to taste

Preparation:
Preheat oven to 400°F (200°C). Line a baking sheet with parchment paper.
Place cod fillets on the prepared baking sheet. Drizzle with olive oil and season with salt and pepper.
In a bowl, mix together breadcrumbs, grated Parmesan cheese, minced garlic, chopped parsley, chopped thyme, salt, and pepper.
Press breadcrumb mixture onto the top of each cod fillet to coat.
Bake in the preheated oven for 12-15 minutes, or until fish is cooked through and topping is golden brown.
Serve hot, garnished with additional chopped herbs if desired.
Prep Time: 25 minutes
Recommended Potassium: 310mg
Phosphorus: 210mg
Sodium: 240mg

Day 23: Mediterranean Chickpea Salad

Ingredients:
1 can (15 ounces) chickpeas, rinsed and drained
1 cucumber, diced
1 cup cherry tomatoes, halved
1/2 cup diced red onion
1/4 cup chopped fresh parsley
Juice of 1 lemon
2 tablespoons olive oil
1 teaspoon dried oregano
Salt and pepper to taste
Crumbled feta cheese for garnish (optional)

Preparation:
In a large bowl, combine chickpeas, diced cucumber, halved cherry tomatoes, diced red onion, and chopped parsley.
In a small bowl, whisk together lemon juice, olive oil, dried oregano, salt, and pepper.
Pour dressing over chickpea salad and toss to coat evenly.
Garnish with crumbled feta cheese if desired.
Serve chilled or at room temperature.
Prep Time: 15 minutes
Recommended Potassium: 440mg
Phosphorus: 125mg
Sodium: 200mg

Day 24: Teriyaki Tofu Stir-Fry

Ingredients:
1 block firm tofu, cubed
2 tablespoons low-sodium soy sauce
2 tablespoons honey
1 tablespoon rice vinegar
1 teaspoon sesame oil
1 tablespoon cornstarch
2 tablespoons olive oil
2 cloves garlic, minced
1 bell pepper, sliced
1 cup broccoli florets
Cooked brown rice for serving

Preparation:
In a bowl, whisk together low-sodium soy sauce, honey, rice vinegar, sesame oil, and cornstarch to make the teriyaki sauce.
Heat olive oil in a large skillet or wok over medium-high heat. Add minced garlic and sauté for 1 minute.
Add cubed tofu to the skillet and cook until browned on all sides.
Add sliced bell pepper and broccoli florets to the skillet. Stir-fry for 3-4 minutes until vegetables are tender-crisp.
Pour teriyaki sauce over the tofu and vegetables. Cook for an additional 2-3 minutes until sauce is thickened.
Serve hot over cooked brown rice.
Prep Time: 30 minutes
Recommended Potassium: 380mg
Phosphorus: 290mg
Sodium: 230mg

Day 25: Spinach and Strawberry Salad with Balsamic Vinaigrette

Ingredients:
4 cups baby spinach leaves
1 cup sliced strawberries
1/4 cup crumbled feta cheese
2 tablespoons chopped almonds
2 tablespoons balsamic vinegar
1 tablespoon olive oil
1 teaspoon honey
Salt and pepper to taste

Preparation:
In a large bowl, combine baby spinach leaves, sliced strawberries, crumbled feta cheese, and chopped almonds.
In a small bowl, whisk together balsamic vinegar, olive oil, honey, salt, and pepper to make the vinaigrette.
Drizzle vinaigrette over the salad and toss gently to coat.
Serve immediately as a refreshing salad.
Prep Time: 10 minutes
Recommended Potassium: 460mg
Phosphorus: 180mg
Sodium: 180mg

Day 26: Lemon Garlic Chicken with Asparagus

Ingredients:
4 boneless, skinless chicken breasts
2 tablespoons olive oil
Zest and juice of 1 lemon
3 cloves garlic, minced

1 tablespoon chopped fresh parsley
Salt and pepper to taste
1 bunch asparagus, trimmed

Preparation:
Preheat oven to 400°F (200°C). Line a baking sheet with parchment paper.
In a bowl, mix together olive oil, lemon zest, lemon juice, minced garlic, chopped parsley, salt, and pepper.
Place chicken breasts on the prepared baking sheet. Arrange asparagus spears around the chicken.
Brush chicken and asparagus with the prepared lemon garlic mixture.
Bake for 20-25 minutes, or until chicken is cooked through and asparagus is tender.
Serve hot, garnished with additional chopped parsley if desired.
Prep Time: 30 minutes
Recommended Potassium: 600mg
Phosphorus: 380mg
Sodium: 210mg

Day 27: Vegetable and Bean Chili

Ingredients:
1 tablespoon olive oil
1 onion, diced
2 cloves garlic, minced
1 bell pepper, diced
1 zucchini, diced
1 cup corn kernels
1 can (15 ounces) kidney beans, drained and rinsed
1 can (15 ounces) black beans, drained and rinsed

1 can (14 ounces) diced tomatoes
2 cups low-sodium vegetable broth
1 tablespoon chili powder
1 teaspoon ground cumin
Salt and pepper to taste
Chopped fresh cilantro for garnish

Preparation:
Heat olive oil in a large pot over medium heat. Add diced onion and minced garlic. Sauté until softened.
Add diced bell pepper, diced zucchini, and corn kernels. Cook for 5-7 minutes until vegetables are tender.
Stir in kidney beans, black beans, diced tomatoes, vegetable broth, chili powder, and ground cumin.
Bring the chili to a simmer and cook for 20-25 minutes, stirring occasionally.
Season with salt and pepper to taste.
Serve hot, garnished with chopped fresh cilantro.
Prep Time: 40 minutes
Recommended Potassium: 770mg
Phosphorus: 410mg
Sodium: 270mg

Day 28: Tofu and Vegetable Curry

Ingredients:
1 block firm tofu, cubed
1 tablespoon olive oil
1 onion, diced
2 cloves garlic, minced
1 tablespoon curry powder
1 teaspoon ground turmeric
1 can (14 ounces) coconut milk

2 cups mixed vegetables (such as bell peppers, carrots, and peas)
Salt and pepper to taste
Cooked rice for serving

Preparation:
Heat olive oil in a large skillet over medium heat. Add diced onion and minced garlic. Sauté until softened.
Add cubed tofu to the skillet and cook until browned.
Stir in curry powder and ground turmeric. Cook for 1-2 minutes until fragrant.
Pour coconut milk into the skillet and bring to a simmer.
Add mixed vegetables and simmer for 10-15 minutes until vegetables are tender and tofu is heated through.
Season with salt and pepper to taste.
Serve hot over cooked rice.
Prep Time: 30 minutes
Recommended Potassium: 550mg
Phosphorus: 280mg
Sodium: 210mg

Day 29: Spinach and Feta Stuffed Chicken Breasts

Ingredients:
4 boneless, skinless chicken breasts
2 cups fresh spinach leaves
1/2 cup crumbled feta cheese
2 cloves garlic, minced
Salt and pepper to taste
1 tablespoon olive oil
Toothpicks or kitchen twine

Preparation:
Preheat oven to 375°F (190°C).
Make a pocket in each chicken breast by cutting a slit horizontally along the side.
In a bowl, mix together fresh spinach leaves, crumbled feta cheese, minced garlic, salt, and pepper.
Stuff each chicken breast with the spinach and feta mixture.
Secure the openings with toothpicks or tie with kitchen twine.
Heat olive oil in an oven-safe skillet over medium-high heat. Add stuffed chicken breasts and sear for 2-3 minutes per side until golden brown.
Transfer skillet to the preheated oven and bake for 20-25 minutes, or until chicken is cooked through.
Remove toothpicks or twine before serving.
Prep Time: 40 minutes
Recommended Potassium: 500mg
Phosphorus: 280mg
Sodium: 220mg

Day 30: Quinoa and Vegetable Stuffed Peppers

Ingredients:
4 large bell peppers, tops removed and seeded
1 cup cooked quinoa
1 cup mixed vegetables (such as corn, peas, carrots, and spinach)
1 can (15 ounces) black beans, drained and rinsed
1 can (14 ounces) diced tomatoes
1 teaspoon ground cumin
1 teaspoon chili powder
Salt and pepper to taste

1/2 cup shredded cheese (optional)

Preparation:
Preheat the oven to 375°F (190°C). Grease a baking dish.
In a large bowl, combine cooked quinoa, mixed vegetables, black beans, diced tomatoes, ground cumin, chili powder, salt, and pepper.
Spoon the quinoa and vegetable mixture into the hollowed-out bell peppers.
Place stuffed peppers in the prepared baking dish. If desired, sprinkle shredded cheese on top.
Cover the baking dish with aluminum foil and bake for 30-35 minutes, or until peppers are tender.
Remove foil and bake for an additional 10 minutes, or until the cheese is melted and bubbly.
Serve hot as a delicious and nutritious meal.
Prep Time: 20 minutes
Recommended Potassium: 770mg
Phosphorus: 200mg
Sodium: 390mg

KIDNEY DISEASES WEEKLY MEAL PLANNER

DATE: _______________

	BREAKFAST	LUNCH	DINNER	SNACKS
MON				
TUE				
WED				
THU				
FRI				
SAT				
SUN				

GROCERY SHOPPING LIST

- ● __________________
- ● __________________
- ● __________________
- ● __________________
- ● __________________

- ● __________________
- ● __________________
- ● __________________
- ● __________________
- ● __________________

- ● __________________
- ● __________________
- ● __________________
- ● __________________
- ● __________________

KIDNEY DISEASES WEEKLY MEAL PLANNER

DATE: _______________

	BREAKFAST	LUNCH	DINNER	SNACKS
MON				
TUE				
WED				
THU				
FRI				
SAT				
SUN				

GROCERY SHOPPING LIST

- ________________
- ________________
- ________________
- ________________
- ________________

- ________________
- ________________
- ________________
- ________________
- ________________

- ________________
- ________________
- ________________
- ________________
- ________________

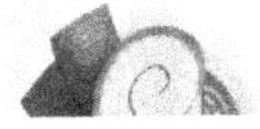
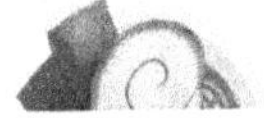

   THE COMPLETE FOODS LISTS FOR KIDNEY DISEAS

KIDNEY DISEASES WEEKLY MEAL PLANNER

DATE: ___________________

	BREAKFAST	LUNCH	DINNER	SNACKS
MON				
TUE				
WED				
THU				
FRI				
SAT				
SUN				

GROCERY SHOPPING LIST

- ____________________
- ____________________
- ____________________
- ____________________
- ____________________

- ____________________
- ____________________
- ____________________
- ____________________
- ____________________

- ____________________
- ____________________
- ____________________
- ____________________
- ____________________

KIDNEY DISEASES WEEKLY MEAL PLANNER

DATE: _______________

	BREAKFAST	LUNCH	DINNER	SNACKS
MON				
TUE				
WED				
THU				
FRI				
SAT				
SUN				

GROCERY SHOPPING LIST

- ________________
- ________________
- ________________
- ________________
- ________________

- ________________
- ________________
- ________________
- ________________
- ________________

- ________________
- ________________
- ________________
- ________________
- ________________

KIDNEY DISEASES WEEKLY MEAL PLANNER

DATE: _______________

	BREAKFAST	LUNCH	DINNER	SNACKS
MON				
TUE				
WED				
THU				
FRI				
SAT				
SUN				

GROCERY SHOPPING LIST

KIDNEY DISEASES WEEKLY MEAL PLANNER

DATE: _______________

	BREAKFAST	LUNCH	DINNER	SNACKS
MON				
TUE				
WED				
THU				
FRI				
SAT				
SUN				

GROCERY SHOPPING LIST

- _______________
- _______________
- _______________
- _______________
- _______________

- _______________
- _______________
- _______________
- _______________
- _______________

- _______________
- _______________
- _______________
- _______________
- _______________

KIDNEY DISEASES WEEKLY MEAL PLANNER

DATE: _______________

	BREAKFAST	LUNCH	DINNER	SNACKS
MON				
TUE				
WED				
THU				
FRI				
SAT				
SUN				

GROCERY SHOPPING LIST

KIDNEY DISEASES WEEKLY MEAL PLANNER

DATE: ___________________

	BREAKFAST	LUNCH	DINNER	SNACKS
MON				
TUE				
WED				
THU				
FRI				
SAT				
SUN				

GROCERY SHOPPING LIST

 THE COMPLETE FOODS LISTS FOR KIDNEY DISEAS

KIDNEY DISEASES WEEKLY MEAL PLANNER

DATE: _______________

	BREAKFAST	LUNCH	DINNER	SNACKS
MON				
TUE				
WED				
THU				
FRI				
SAT				
SUN				

GROCERY SHOPPING LIST

- ______________
- ______________
- ______________
- ______________
- ______________

- ______________
- ______________
- ______________
- ______________
- ______________

- ______________
- ______________
- ______________
- ______________
- ______________

KIDNEY DISEASES WEEKLY MEAL PLANNER

DATE: _______________

	BREAKFAST	LUNCH	DINNER	SNACKS
MON				
TUE				
WED				
THU				
FRI				
SAT				
SUN				

GROCERY SHOPPING LIST

KIDNEY DISEASES WEEKLY MEAL PLANNER

DATE: _______________

	BREAKFAST	LUNCH	DINNER	SNACKS
MON				
TUE				
WED				
THU				
FRI				
SAT				
SUN				

GROCERY SHOPPING LIST

- ____________________
- ____________________
- ____________________
- ____________________
- ____________________

- ____________________
- ____________________
- ____________________
- ____________________
- ____________________

- ____________________
- ____________________
- ____________________
- ____________________
- ____________________

KIDNEY DISEASES WEEKLY MEAL PLANNER

DATE: _______________

	BREAKFAST	LUNCH	DINNER	SNACKS
MON				
TUE				
WED				
THU				
FRI				
SAT				
SUN				

GROCERY SHOPPING LIST

  THE COMPLETE FOODS LISTS FOR KIDNEY DISEAS

KIDNEY DISEASES WEEKLY MEAL PLANNER

DATE: _______________

	BREAKFAST	LUNCH	DINNER	SNACKS
MON				
TUE				
WED				
THU				
FRI				
SAT				
SUN				

GROCERY SHOPPING LIST

- _______________
- _______________
- _______________
- _______________
- _______________

- _______________
- _______________
- _______________
- _______________
- _______________

- _______________
- _______________
- _______________
- _______________
- _______________

KIDNEY DISEASES WEEKLY MEAL PLANNER

DATE: _______________

	BREAKFAST	LUNCH	DINNER	SNACKS
MON				
TUE				
WED				
THU				
FRI				
SAT				
SUN				

GROCERY SHOPPING LIST

- _______________
- _______________
- _______________
- _______________
- _______________

- _______________
- _______________
- _______________
- _______________
- _______________

- _______________
- _______________
- _______________
- _______________
- _______________

THE COMPLETE FOODS LISTS FOR KIDNEY DISEAS

KIDNEY DISEASES WEEKLY MEAL PLANNER

DATE: _______________

	BREAKFAST	LUNCH	DINNER	SNACKS
MON				
TUE				
WED				
THU				
FRI				
SAT				
SUN				

GROCERY SHOPPING LIST

KIDNEY DISEASES WEEKLY MEAL PLANNER

DATE: _______________

	BREAKFAST	LUNCH	DINNER	SNACKS
MON				
TUE				
WED				
THU				
FRI				
SAT				
SUN				

GROCERY SHOPPING LIST

KIDNEY DISEASES WEEKLY MEAL PLANNER

DATE: _______________

	BREAKFAST	LUNCH	DINNER	SNACKS
MON				
TUE				
WED				
THU				
FRI				
SAT				
SUN				

GROCERY SHOPPING LIST

KIDNEY DISEASES WEEKLY MEAL PLANNER

DATE: _______________

	BREAKFAST	LUNCH	DINNER	SNACKS
MON				
TUE				
WED				
THU				
FRI				
SAT				
SUN				

GROCERY SHOPPING LIST

- ● _______________
- ● _______________
- ● _______________
- ● _______________
- ● _______________

- ● _______________
- ● _______________
- ● _______________
- ● _______________
- ● _______________

- ● _______________
- ● _______________
- ● _______________
- ● _______________
- ● _______________

THE COMPLETE FOODS LISTS FOR KIDNEY DISEAS

KIDNEY DISEASES WEEKLY MEAL PLANNER

DATE: ___________________

	BREAKFAST	LUNCH	DINNER	SNACKS
MON				
TUE				
WED				
THU				
FRI				
SAT				
SUN				

GROCERY SHOPPING LIST

- ________________
- ________________
- ________________
- ________________
- ________________

- ________________
- ________________
- ________________
- ________________
- ________________

- ________________
- ________________
- ________________
- ________________
- ________________

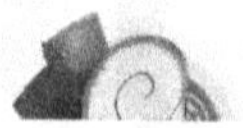
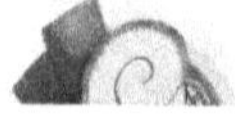

KIDNEY DISEASES WEEKLY MEAL PLANNER

DATE: _______________

	BREAKFAST	LUNCH	DINNER	SNACKS
MON				
TUE				
WED				
THU				
FRI				
SAT				
SUN				

GROCERY SHOPPING LIST

    THE COMPLETE FOODS LISTS FOR KIDNEY DISEAS

KIDNEY DISEASES WEEKLY MEAL PLANNER

DATE: _______________

	BREAKFAST	LUNCH	DINNER	SNACKS
MON				
TUE				
WED				
THU				
FRI				
SAT				
SUN				

GROCERY SHOPPING LIST

KIDNEY DISEASES WEEKLY MEAL PLANNER

DATE: _______________

	BREAKFAST	LUNCH	DINNER	SNACKS
MON				
TUE				
WED				
THU				
FRI				
SAT				
SUN				

GROCERY SHOPPING LIST

KIDNEY DISEASES WEEKLY MEAL PLANNER

DATE: ______________

	BREAKFAST	LUNCH	DINNER	SNACKS
MON				
TUE				
WED				
THU				
FRI				
SAT				
SUN				

GROCERY SHOPPING LIST

- ___________
- ___________
- ___________
- ___________
- ___________

- ___________
- ___________
- ___________
- ___________
- ___________

- ___________
- ___________
- ___________
- ___________
- ___________

KIDNEY DISEASES WEEKLY MEAL PLANNER

DATE: _______________

	BREAKFAST	LUNCH	DINNER	SNACKS
MON				
TUE				
WED				
THU				
FRI				
SAT				
SUN				

GROCERY SHOPPING LIST

KIDNEY DISEASES WEEKLY MEAL PLANNER

DATE: _______________

	BREAKFAST	LUNCH	DINNER	SNACKS
MON				
TUE				
WED				
THU				
FRI				
SAT				
SUN				

GROCERY SHOPPING LIST

KIDNEY DISEASES WEEKLY MEAL PLANNER

DATE: ______________

	BREAKFAST	LUNCH	DINNER	SNACKS
MON				
TUE				
WED				
THU				
FRI				
SAT				
SUN				

GROCERY SHOPPING LIST

KIDNEY DISEASES WEEKLY MEAL PLANNER

DATE: _______________

	BREAKFAST	LUNCH	DINNER	SNACKS
MON				
TUE				
WED				
THU				
FRI				
SAT				
SUN				

GROCERY SHOPPING LIST

- ______________
- ______________
- ______________
- ______________
- ______________

- ______________
- ______________
- ______________
- ______________
- ______________

- ______________
- ______________
- ______________
- ______________
- ______________

KIDNEY DISEASES WEEKLY MEAL PLANNER

DATE: ___________________

	BREAKFAST	LUNCH	DINNER	SNACKS
MON				
TUE				
WED				
THU				
FRI				
SAT				
SUN				

GROCERY SHOPPING LIST

- ________________
- ________________
- ________________
- ________________
- ________________

- ________________
- ________________
- ________________
- ________________
- ________________

- ________________
- ________________
- ________________
- ________________
- ________________

     THE COMPLETE FOODS LISTS FOR KIDNEY DISEAS

KIDNEY DISEASES WEEKLY MEAL PLANNER

DATE: _______________

	BREAKFAST	LUNCH	DINNER	SNACKS
MON				
TUE				
WED				
THU				
FRI				
SAT				
SUN				

GROCERY SHOPPING LIST

- ________________
- ________________
- ________________
- ________________
- ________________

- ________________
- ________________
- ________________
- ________________
- ________________

- ________________
- ________________
- ________________
- ________________
- ________________

KIDNEY DISEASES WEEKLY MEAL PLANNER

DATE: _______________

	BREAKFAST	LUNCH	DINNER	SNACKS
MON				
TUE				
WED				
THU				
FRI				
SAT				
SUN				

GROCERY SHOPPING LIST

- ___________
- ___________
- ___________
- ___________
- ___________

- ___________
- ___________
- ___________
- ___________
- ___________

- ___________
- ___________
- ___________
- ___________
- ___________

THE COMPLETE FOODS LISTS FOR KIDNEY DISEAS

My Valued Reader,

I trust this culinary journey has not only ignited your passion for wholesome eating but has also become a haven of inspiration, solace, and invaluable insights. Each carefully curated recipe within this kidney diseases food list reflects a dedication to excellence, with a profound understanding of the comprehensive guide to the kidney diseases diet.

Crafted with meticulous attention to detail, these recipes go beyond the realm of mere sustenance; they are a testament to the art of nourishing the body and soul.

Your reviews, experiences, and insights are needed to guide me on improving this book.

Every evaluation is a stepping stone for refinement, as I aspire to tailor this food list to surpass your expectations. Let's engage in a dialogue that transcends the pages, creating a connection that resonates with your culinary preferences and well-being goals.

Warm Culinary Regards,

Tina Feldman

Conclusion

In conclusion, understanding and implementing dietary changes are essential aspects of managing kidney disease effectively. The comprehensive foods lists provided for kidney disease offer a valuable resource for individuals seeking to make informed choices about their nutrition. By embracing whole and minimally processed foods, incorporating kidney-friendly ingredients, and being mindful of potassium, phosphorus, and sodium levels, individuals with kidney disease can take proactive steps towards improving their health and well-being.

Moreover, adopting cooking techniques tailored to reduce sodium and phosphorus content in meals further empowers individuals to create flavorful dishes without compromising their dietary restrictions. From selecting low-sodium ingredients to employing cooking methods that minimize phosphorus absorption, these strategies contribute to a kidney-friendly lifestyle that promotes optimal kidney function and overall health.

It is important to recognize that dietary needs may vary depending on the stage of kidney disease and individual health considerations. Therefore, consulting with a healthcare professional or registered dietitian is highly recommended to tailor dietary recommendations to specific needs and goals.